T0339859

# HOW TO LIVE WELL WITH DEMENTIA

*How to Live Well with Dementia: Expert Help for People Living with Dementia and their Family, Friends, and Care Partners* provides an array of essential guidance about the different aspects of dementia for all whose lives are touched by dementia, including people living with dementia and their support network.

Following an effective Q&A framework, this book offers valuable, easy-to-navigate guidance on the burning questions that those living with a dementia diagnosis and their carer/supporter need to know. Questions addressed include 'How can I adjust to life with the diagnosis?', 'How can I plan for the future?', and 'How can we support our loved ones living with dementia?'. It provides expert explanations about changes in the brain and the various causes and types of dementia, as well as support on how to adjust to living with a diagnosis. It also offers practical information about care planning and advanced directives, maintaining health and social connections, accessing appropriate community care, and supporting medical and hospital care. It concludes with important self-care information for care/support partners.

Written jointly by academic experts and experts through lived experience, this book is indispensable for people living with dementia, care partners, and anyone wanting to understand more about the condition, as well as health and social care professionals and students of health and social care.

**Anthea Innes** moved from Scotland to Canada in 2022, where she is a professor of health, ageing, and society; Gilbrea research chair in ageing and mental health; and director of the Gilbrea Centre for Studies in Aging at McMaster University. She has conducted social research on dementia for nearly 30 years.

**Megan E. O'Connell** is a registered doctoral psychologist and a professor of psychology at the University of Saskatchewan, Saskatchewan, Canada. She leads the clinical neuropsychology team in the diagnostic Rural and Remote Memory Clinic, provides care partner support, and researches issues related to dementia care.

**Carmel Geoghegan** is based in Ireland and was primary carer for her mother who lived with mixed dementia. She has remained an advocate and supporter of campaigns that keep the spotlight on dementia and end-of-life care. Her priority is the development of practices and policies that respect people living with a dementia diagnosis, particularly in rural areas.

**Phyllis Fehr** is a person living with dementia in Canada. She is currently a patient advisory to the Alzheimer's Board for Canada. She provides local leadership to the Empowering Dementia-Friendly Communities Hamilton, Haldimand project, and has written and spoken about her experiences nationally and internationally.

# BPS ASK THE EXPERTS IN PSYCHOLOGY SERIES

## British Psychological Society

Routledge, in partnership with the British Psychological Society (BPS), is pleased to present BPS Ask the Experts, a new popular science series that addresses key issues and answers the burning questions. Drawing on the expertise of established psychologists, every book in the series provides authoritative and straightforward guidance on pressing topics that matter to real people in their everyday lives.

All books in the BPS Ask the Experts series are written for the reader with no prior knowledge or experience. For answers to everything you ever wanted to know about issues important to you, ask the expert!

### Managing Your Gaming and Social Media Habits
From Science to Solutions
*Catherine Knibbs*

### How to Live Well with Dementia
Expert Help for People Living with Dementia and their Family, Friends, and Care Partners
*Anthea Innes, Megan E. O'Connell, Carmel Geoghegan, and Phyllis Fehr*

For more information about this series, please visit: https://www.routledge.com/our-products/book-series/BPSATE

# HOW TO LIVE WELL WITH DEMENTIA

## EXPERT HELP FOR PEOPLE LIVING WITH DEMENTIA AND THEIR FAMILY, FRIENDS, AND CARE PARTNERS

Anthea Innes, Megan E. O'Connell,
Carmel Geoghegan, and Phyllis Fehr

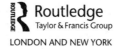

Routledge
Taylor & Francis Group

LONDON AND NEW YORK

Designed cover image: getty images

First published 2025
by Routledge
4 Park Square, Milton Park, Abingdon, Oxon OX14 4RN

and by Routledge
605 Third Avenue, New York, NY 10158

*Routledge is an imprint of the Taylor & Francis Group, an informa business*

*British Library Cataloguing-in-Publication Data*
A catalogue record for this book is available from the British Library

ISBN: 9781032599991 (hbk)
ISBN: 9781032599977 (pbk)
ISBN: 9781003457138 (ebk)

DOI: 10.4324/9781003457138

Typeset in Bembo
by Deanta Global Publishing Services, Chennai, India

# CONTENTS

# FOREWORD

As the CEO of the Alzheimer Society of Canada, it's my privilege to introduce this remarkable book authored by Anthea Innes, Megan O'Connell, Carmel Geoghegan, and Phyllis Fehr. Their collective wisdom and diverse experiences have culminated in a guide that promises support for those navigating the complexities of dementia.

Dementia, with its myriad challenges and uncertainties, touches the lives of millions worldwide. This book is a roadmap, meticulously crafted to traverse the journey of dementia. From the initial steps of diagnosis to the pivotal moments of transition and caregiving, each chapter illuminates the path forward with clarity and compassion. What emerges is a holistic approach that acknowledges the unique experiences of each individual while providing a framework for collective understanding and support.

For those facing dementia, whether personally or as a caregiver, this book offers practical advice and heartfelt encouragement. And for healthcare professionals, it serves as a valuable resource, enriching their understanding and guiding their practice towards more compassionate care.

As we delve into these pages, let us recognize that dementia isn't merely a medical issue; it's a journey that affects emotions, reshapes connections, and demands unity. May this book be a practical guide, lighting the way towards a better future for all impacted by dementia.

*Christopher Barry,*
*CEO, Alzheimer Society of Canada*

# INTRODUCTION

This book is co-authored by four people. Our introduction reflects the order of the names as they appear on the front cover. This does not reflect any order of value of the contributions each author has made. It is our collective experiences and reflections, we believe, that has enabled us to create a collection of chapters seeking to help the person with the diagnosis and their family, friends, and care partners, to live well with their journey with dementia.

Anthea Innes is a social scientist who has been researching the social aspects of dementia since 1996 (over 25 years). At the core of her work has been a concern to hear the views and experiences of those directly impacted by dementia: the person diagnosed, their family and other supporters, and paid workers. Megan O'Connell is a clinical psychologist who has been working directly with people living with dementia for around 25 years, including in a memory clinic where people are diagnosed and supported throughout their journey with dementia, as well as conducting research about dementia. Carmel Geoghegan began caring for her mother who was diagnosed with dementia in 2011. Although her mother has since died, she has continued to be involved in community work to support people living with dementia and their family members and supporters. She set up Dementia Ireland Empowering Communities in 2017 and has been active in promoting better support and care for people living with dementia in her home country of Ireland, and internationally. Phyllis Fehr has been living with dementia for the last 16 years, although the first few years were without the diagnosis as she worked her way through the diagnostic process. Phyllis has been involved at national level in Canada, as well as internationally, sharing her experiences of living with dementia to create awareness of the condition and to promote better support for those with the diagnosis. It is from these collective experiences that we have worked together to create this book with the intention of offering help to people living with dementia, their family and friends, and care partners.

This book is intended as a guide for general readers who may be experiencing dementia as a person diagnosed with dementia, or a family or friend who is providing support and care for someone living with dementia. It also works as a general guide for health and social care staff to understanding dementia and enabling them to think about how best to support the person living with dementia. It focuses on the key points in the journey with dementia and how best to support people living with dementia and their care partners as their journey with dementia progresses.

The book is organized into three parts. Part 1 has three chapters. The first chapter is a longer chapter as it considers the process of getting a diagnosis and the multitude of common questions that individuals often have as they seek to understand what dementia is and what it means for them. Two shorter chapters then consider how people begin to adjust to living with the diagnosis and how they might begin to plan for the future.

Part 2 focuses on what happens after the diagnosis and how to live well with dementia. This is the time in the journey with dementia when the person living with dementia is living at home in the community. The first chapter in Part 2 (Chapter 4) discusses how to maintain social health and well-being. Chapter 5 moves on to consider the questions that are often asked about how to access care and support in the community. People living with dementia will often require hospital appointments and perhaps admissions, as part of their dementia care or for other health issues, and Chapter 6 aims to address the common questions that people have about how best to support the person living with dementia with hospital appointments and admissions.

Part 3 focuses on the part of the journey with dementia when transitions may be necessary. Chapter 7 discusses a point that many find difficult to consider and then implement – planning a move to long-term care. Another difficult transition can be when palliative care is introduced and when end-of-life care is required, this is the topic of Chapter 8. Chapter 9, the final chapter, seeks to directly answer questions about the needs of care partners and supporters. Here, we consider the very important topic of care partners 'looking after yourself'.

While we recognize that the chapters may be a false division in relation to different individuals' experiences, we have organized the book in this way to reflect the progression of the journey of living with dementia and supporting a person living with dementia. For many, the diagnosis and adjustment part of the journey can take many years due to accessing diagnostic services and perhaps having 'minor' symptoms (Part 1). Sometimes, an individual's journey might progress quickly from diagnosis (Part 1) to the need for long-term care or end-of-life care (Part 3). For others, 'living with dementia' (Part 2) will span many years and different supports might be required at different moments in time. We fully acknowledge that the journey of each individual living with dementia, their families, and supporters will be unique to their circumstances. However, the chapters in this book discuss different parts of the journey that are common to many and provide a way to identify an issue that might be of concern at a particular moment in time. Individually, the chapters provide a 'drop-in' opportunity to reflect and hopefully find some suggestions that may be of assistance as an individual with dementia or a family member or support is traversing the journey of life with dementia.

# Part 1

# 1

---

# DOES SOMETHING FEEL DIFFERENT? IS IT TIME TO SEEK A DIAGNOSIS?

## WHEN DO I WORRY ABOUT CHANGES IN THINKING – WHAT IS THE EXPECTED AGEING OF THE BRAIN AND THINKING?

We all experience lapses in memory – we go into a room and forget why we went in there. We forget the names of people we know we have met, many of us rely on some sort of assistance to remind us of what we need from the grocery store, and most of us keep track of appointments in some sort of calendar system because if we do not, we will forget. We forget who we told stories to and find ourselves repeating stories to the same people. Most of the time we can brush off these memory lapses as part of the human experience. Many of us are aware that memory is less efficient as we advance in age (Salthouse, 2010). We reassure ourselves that these lapses are part of normal ageing. At some point, however, these lapses become more common and make it hard to accomplish what we need to do daily – and at this point we ask ourselves: ok, is this when we need to worry?

As we age, we also experience changes in language. Most commonly, we know a word but can't quite access it; it is the frustrating tip of the tongue – we know it is there, but we just can't seem

DOI: 10.4324/9781003457138-2

to grab it, only for the word to come to us several hours later. The efficiency in accessing facts from our mental library of facts (semantic memory network) commonly declines with expected and typical ageing changes in thinking, also referred to as cognition. This *tip of the tongue* phenomenon is so common, we see it in many of our friends and family who are middle-aged or older (Abrams & Davis, 2016). At some point, accessing the word we want to say makes it hard to get through a conversation without halting and searching for words, or sometimes we say the wrong word, and we ask ourselves: ok, is this when we need to worry?

Hopefully, these examples illustrate how hard it can be to separate worrisome changes in thinking or cognition versus those we expect to happen with expected and typical cognitive ageing. After the childhood/adolescent stage of brain development ceases in the early to mid twenties, brain maturation is associated with two main processes: (1) brain-based changes that can be simplistically summarized as an accumulation of damage that results in cell death or disrupted communication within the brain and (2) continued learning of new information and stimulation that result in the formation of new connections in the brain (Salthouse, 2010). In fact, when you have learnt new information and can recall this information after a delay, you have made a new connection in your brain called 'long-term potentiation'. Contrary to what might have been taught even as recently as a decade ago, we know that humans grow new brain cells through our lifespan and some of these new brain cells are related to memory (neurogenesis in the hippocampal formation) (Goncalves et al., 2016). Much of the decades of research on the development of the brain in adulthood to older adulthood has, however, focused on the consequences of accumulated brain-based dysfunction, which we refer to as normal cognitive ageing.

Cognitive ageing has been studied by looking at the same people as they advance in age over decades (longitudinally) and by comparing people measured once who are of different ages (cross-sectionally). Regardless of the method used to measure cognitive ageing or regardless of the sample studied, some cognitive processes appear to increase as we age. Specifically, our knowledge of the meaning of words (our accumulated vocabulary) increases until our seventies. However, most cognitive processes appear to decrease after our twenties. Our speed of mental thinking, which is closely linked to our ability to mentally track more than one task at the same time, decreases with advancing age. Our efficiency in learning and retaining new information (episodic memory), our ability to understand our visual and spatial world, and our complex reasoning abilities also decline with advancing age (Salthouse, 2010). It is not all bad news – when compared with younger adults, older adults are more likely to use more information when making a decision, which some have labelled 'wisdom' (Worthy et al., 2011).

Phyllis reflects on her early concerns that 'something' was not 'quite right':

This is a very hard question to answer, as in the beginning, the changes are mild and you may not notice them. For me, in the beginning I was having trouble with writing; documentation was a problem that I was having but I was unaware of it. Being a nurse, documentation was highly important, but it was taking longer and longer to do and was taking up more of my day. It started to interfere with my Physical Therapy (PT) care. My practice changed and I made sure my PT care came first, then when I had time, I would do my documentation. As this progressed, my documentation started happening after the shift was over and it was taking longer to do. At this time, I didn't realize what was happening. It wasn't until other things started to rear their ugly heads that I realized I was having a problem. If I looked at each thing separately, it wasn't a big deal. But when you combine them and look at the bigger picture, oh my, that's when I knew I had a problem. Some of the other things that were happening were having trouble multitasking, being unable to remember how to mix a drug, and having to take the time to look it up. Safety was always key for me, so taking the time to research something didn't bother me, but again there is more time being taken out of my day. I also started to notice things in my personal life going out of 'wack', but that didn't matter to me at the time as it really didn't harm anyone or anything. It wasn't until I took the time to look at the whole picture that I realized I had a problem and called the doctor.

While waiting for my doctor's appointment, I took stock of my life. Is there anything I can do to make things better? At the time, I was working two jobs, maybe I was overdoing it? I personally didn't think I was, but I let one job go. I thought, maybe I was just tired. When I finally saw the doctor, I was left feeling like I was crazy, that there was nothing wrong with me. This ended up being a very long process for me as the doctor believed I was fine. With continued pressure from me, he started to check for medical reasons for my symptoms. Could it be the menopause? Depression? Metabolic disorders? But all the tests were negative and when I brought up the possibility of dementia, he ignored it. Now what? What should I do? I was starting to become very concerned and took a leave of absence from work. This is when I saw other things happening like being irritable and short-tempered. Maybe not due to the dementia process, but due to frustration, and feeling like I was not being heard. I eventually saw my doctor again and told a lie, as I knew a neurologist would understand and may be more willing to look into it, so I said my migraines had returned and he quickly sent me off to see a neurologist. And, yes! This is when things started to change for me. I was being heard. Tests were ordered, referrals were made. It took five years, but finally, I did receive a diagnosis and I knew I wasn't going crazy. I knew all along what I was looking at because I saw signs in me that I had seen in my own mother and grandmother, both of whom had Alzheimer's.

## WHEN SHOULD WE SEE A HEALTHCARE PROVIDER?

If we should expect changes in memory like forgetting who you told a story to last week and repeating yourself as part of expected cognitive ageing, when should we begin to worry that this is something else? Forgetting over the span of days is common, but forgetting over the span of hours might be a more worrisome sign. Occasional worrisome signs are not likely to be of concern. Occasional worrisome memory lapses can be the result of attentional lapses – if we are distracted either by internal thoughts or by something in our environment – they can look like a memory problem, but they are more of an attentional problem. Memory is like a bank – to get money out of it, you must put money into it in the first place. Not paying attention is like not putting money in the bank – no wonder you could not get anything out of the bank, you didn't have anything in there in the first place!

If, however, memory lapses are common, or if they impact your ability to do your daily tasks, it might be a good idea to see a healthcare provider. Expected changes in thinking associated with advanced age, called cognitive ageing, can make it difficult to tell when there is a brain-based disease (like those causing dementia) present. If we expect you to have problems learning and retaining new information due to advancing age as part of cognitive ageing, how can we tell if you have memory problems? When psychologists or neuropsychologists (specialists in brain–behaviour relations) measure cognition, they frequently compare a person's performance to their age-matched peers – this method allows us to determine, for example, if that person's performance on tests of memory is expected given their age (O'Connell et al., 2021).

Cognitive screening tests are not typically adjusted for age, rather these are tests where most people tend to do well and when people do not do well it suggests that further assessment is warranted. These methods of assessment are not perfect – sometimes people who have a brain-based disease do very well on these cognitive tests, and sometimes people do poorly on these cognitive tests because of factors outside of brain diseases. These tests tend to have the core assumptions that the people taking the tests are similar in cultural, linguistic, and educational background to those who were first studied when the tests were developed. More research is needed in how to accurately assess cognition with linguistic and cultural diversity and with those who have varying experience with formal education (Franzen et al., 2020).

Cognitive assessments are only a small part of the diagnostic process to investigate brain-based diseases. Foremost, a full medical workup is required. If our body is very ill, it can impact the functioning of our brain (Mattison, 2020). As we age, we are more likely to experience problems with the functioning of our brain due to problems with our health. For example, it is common for untreated bladder infections to result in changes in the behaviour and thinking of older adults, and the treatment for this is to treat the illness – the bladder infection. In addition to a full medical workup to rule out health conditions that could be impacting the functioning of the brain, a clinical history and an interview with someone who knows the person well is part of the diagnostic process.

## WHAT HAPPENS IF I CAN'T GET MY HEALTHCARE PROVIDER TO TAKE MY WORRIES SERIOUSLY?

Unfortunately, some people experience resistance from their primary healthcare provider when they bring up their worries about their changes in thinking, for example, frequent memory lapses. It is possible that you do not have access to the same primary healthcare provider and every time you visit a physician or nurse, you have to see someone new and explain your medical history again. Or it is possible that your primary care provider who has known you for many years keeps reassuring you that the worries you have are changes we all experience as we advance in age. People who present with symptoms before the age of 65, also referred to as young onset dementia, can experience challenges convincing their primary care providers that something is wrong, in part because it is so unexpected (O'Connell et al., 2014). Recall, expected cognitive ageing is associated with numerous declines in thinking performance apart from acquired vocabulary knowledge (Salthouse, 2010), and it is possible that the primary care provider is correct – the numerous examples of memory lapses are consistent with what we would expect from normal ageing. For some people, subjective cognitive concerns or subjective memory concerns are just that – you think you have a problem but when you get assessed, your cognition is consistent with what we would expect from your peers. It is possible that you feel your concerns about cognition were too hastily categorized as subjective cognitive impairment – what do you do then? Keep seeking help and ask for referrals.

Anecdotally, we have witnessed that many people experiencing brain-based cognitive changes spend years brushing off their concerns and would prefer to deny that there is anything wrong. Frequently, their family feels the same – there is a noticeable lapse, but they talk themselves out of worrying, suggesting that there is likely a good explanation for it. At some point, however, it is undeniable that a decline has occurred. It is usually at this point that people should begin to mention concerns to their primary care provider – and this is often years into the process of change. Still, many families have to act as advocates and convince their primary care provider to make a referral to a speciality clinic for a diagnosis (Morgan et al., 2014). How does one act as an advocate? Be informed about the symptoms that matter to the person/the family (e.g. memory lapses) and the consequences for daily functioning (e.g. forgetting to pay bills), recruit help from people known to the family and who know the person living with dementia well and can report on what they have observed – maybe even bring them to appointments. And most of all – be persistent. It is possible to seek a different healthcare provider to get a referral. Sometimes, even a speciality memory clinic is unable to make a clear diagnosis, but the clinic follows people over time – comparing a person's current cognitive performance to their performance a year ago is better than comparing a person's performance to their peers.

In Ireland, especially in rural areas, it is still very much a diagnosis with a very outdated label attached. It is not yet fully accepted as a disease like any other that with the right treatment, supports, and community understanding a person can live a very full, active, and functioning life. They can still be very much part of their community. If people are diagnosed early they can remain at work, maybe not in their present position, but may move to a less demanding role. Many general practitioners (GPs) are still very much of the thinking that they are protecting the person, when in fact they are denying them a better quality of life. There is also a practice of treating the obvious symptoms such as depression and not looking more closely at underlying issues. Many GPs put memory issues down to the 'ageing process'. We have to change this thinking, and this can only be achieved by more informed education and understanding of what dementia is and how the brain is affected.

Over the past number of years, we have been engaging with various disciplines within the medical training programmes. This has been a fascinating experience as many experienced medical staff, i.e. a community nurse, would not have encountered patients with an early diagnosis or younger members of the community (Health Service Executive, 2023). They are shocked when they see my colleague who is living with Alzheimer's, has been diagnosed for over ten years, and is still very vocal in advocating for a change in health policies (Kumari, 2023). It is also important to recognize that some medications have side effects, and this manifests differently in each individual. Brain fog is a common side effect of many prescription drugs.

It is important to follow up with your healthcare provider and if you need to bring a trusted friend to support you at the consultation, please do so. Most healthcare providers will listen, so never give up and insist on a referral.

Carmel reflects on how the diagnosis of her mother came about:

My own experience with my Mum: she had been diagnosed with osteoporosis by her clinicians due to having had many falls over a number of years. However, years later she was finally diagnosed with mixed dementia, vascular/frontotemporal, but Mum was nearing the end of her journey with dementia by then. Additionally, Mum had been medicated to a point that was over the legal recommended dosage of antidepressants, as she had also been diagnosed with depression. The symptoms of depression would no doubt manifest if you are in fear of losing your mind and afraid to mention or acknowledge that you are experiencing some difficulties. Also, living in the West of Ireland, due to weather and social/rural isolation, depression is often a health issue and not uncommon for people to experience.

I believe that if my Mum had originally been thoroughly examined, referred, and correctly diagnosed, she would probably have lived a very different last ten years of her life.

## WHAT IS HAPPENING IN THE BRAIN? – CAUSES OF DEMENTIA

Dementia is a term we use to refer to different symptoms of cognitive impairment. The cognitive impairment must be a decline from previous functioning, and for this reason, diagnosing dementia in persons with intellectual disability, such as due to Down syndrome, typically requires following people over time. We need to assess to the best of our abilities what the person's cognitive status was prior to the onset of cognitive difficulties. For example, did they always have trouble with learning and retaining new information? This assessment involves an understanding of early development, educational attainment, and any educational difficulties, occupational history, and hobbies. In addition, cognitive tests where performance tends to hold even when diseases of the brain are present are used to help estimate cognitive function prior to the current changes that led the family to seek help (Overman et al., 2021). For a diagnosis of dementia using the most recent diagnostic manual for mental disorders (where the term 'major neurocognitive disorder' is used), there must be evidence of problems with memory and another area of cognition such as language, understanding one's visual-spatial world, the integration of what you perceive from your senses with movement, the ability to pay attention to complex information, the ability to understand the social impact of one's behaviour, and the ability to organize, sequence, plan, and coordinate all other cognitive abilities, which is sometimes referred to as executive function (American Psychiatric Association, 2022). The impairment in cognition must be of sufficient severity to stop one from doing one's daily tasks without help; and commonly these are complicated daily tasks like managing medications or appointments, managing finances, driving, and even figuring out the complex remote controls for TVs. Cognitive problems that are not as severe and might not result in as many problems functioning independently in daily life are diagnosed as mild cognitive impairment (MCI) or 'mild neurocognitive disorder' (American Psychiatric Association, 2022). Some people with mild cognitive impairment are diagnosed at the earliest stages of a more severe disease, such as Alzheimer's disease (AD), which could be supported by the presence of a high amyloid burden from neuroimaging or other biomarker sources. However, for other people, a diagnosis might require tracking them over time.

*Vascular dementia.* Dementia can be caused by various brain-based diseases, and most of these progressively cause brain cell death. The progressive nature of most of these brain-based diseases means that cognitive and functional impairments worsen over time and the need for care tends to increase. Which aspects of cognition a person has difficulties with depends on where in the brain the disease tends to start. Strokes can impact almost any circuit in the brain, but certain areas are more likely, such as the small arteries feeding the memory system. Repeated strokes can cause vascular dementia, as can 'silent' or smaller strokes in the connection systems of the brain. Transient ischemic attacks (TIAs) are similar to small strokes but differ predominantly in that symptoms resolve with TIAs, whereas strokes have residual symptoms. Some small strokes in small vessels cause bleeds, or strokes can interact with other brain diseases (e.g. Alzheimer's disease), and dementia can be caused by more than one disease (Korczyn, 2002). Vascular dementia is sometimes misdiagnosed or just not detected because having mini stokes can often result in a fall, sustaining a breakage in a bone (fracture) (Ruggiero et al., 2024). This is the main focus on admittance to hospital and if osteoporosis is diagnosed as the reason for the fracture, any further investigation may cease.

*Alzheimer's disease.* Although many specialists argue that dementia due to multiple diseases is the most common cause, dementia due to Alzheimer's disease is frequently described as the most common disease underlying dementia. Dementia due to Alzheimer's disease is typically associated with cell death in the areas of the brain responsible for learning and retaining new information (episodic memory in the hippocampal formation inside each temporal lobe). Dementia due to Alzheimer's disease progresses to impact our understanding of our visual-spatial world, including spatial navigation and the retrieval of information from our networks of fact-based knowledge (semantic memory network), which can impact language. Complex attention (alternating attention between two tasks or paying attention to more than one thing at a time) and executive function are also impacted relatively early in the disease process (Allain et al., 2013). Behaviour problems commonly reported include lack of interest in engaging in any activities in the absence of sad mood (i.e. apathy vs depression)

(Nobis & Husain, 2018). Additionally, people with memory problems often believe that others have come into their home and stolen or moved lost items, and sometimes people with profound memory problems can fill in the gaps by telling stories that others do not agree happened (confabulation) (El Haj et al., 2020). In the most severe forms of the disease, global cognitive impairment and problems with basic functions like swallowing are common in persons living with AD. Although cell death could impact the brain circuits responsible for respiration and heart rate, typically people living with severely progressed AD die of other causes like a viral infection or bacterial pneumonia (Todd et al., 2013). Cell death in AD is noticeable by the presence of beta-amyloid plaques and neurofibrillary tangles (from phosphorylated tau or p-tau), and recent advances in neuroimaging and (very soon to be more widely integrated into clinical use) blood-based biomarkers allow for the quantification of the amount of beta-amyloid and p-tau in the brain, leading many speciality clinics to use this as a diagnostic aid for Alzheimer's disease (Teunissen et al., 2022). As less invasive mechanisms for biomarkers, such as blood-based or saliva-based methods for reliably and accurately detecting AD biomarkers, become readily available in the near future, we predict that diagnostic processes will require biomarker support (see the biological research framework of AD [Jack et al., 2018] and, as of writing this book, the framework is in the process of being updated). However, it will be challenging to ensure that all regions of the world have the resources available to measure biomarkers to avoid creating further disparities in diagnostic access than currently exist.

*Parkinson's disease.* A different type of cell death is associated with Parkinson's disease (PD), which impacts deep structures in the brain responsible for motor control (Lewy bodies in the substantia nigra – Lewy bodies refer to how the cells look after they die). Dementia due to Parkinson's disease begins with a constellation of motor control challenges that characterize PD, such as resting tremor, muscles that do not relax and tend to stay rigid, problems with walking and balance, slowed movement and thinking, reduced movement usually seen in reduced arm swing or loss of movement in facial muscles, small handwriting, loss of smell – but there are many causes for this, depression, and a specific type of sleep dysfunction (acting out one's dreams). When the cognitive difficulties progress to include memory and executive function problems, a diagnosis of dementia due to PD might be warranted. People can live for many years with PD and not have dementia due to PD, and sometimes they die of other causes before being diagnosed with dementia (Lethbridge et al., 2013).

*Lewy body dementia.* Sometimes, sleep dysfunction and cognitive problems are present at the same time as some of the motor symptoms, albeit less severe rigidity and tremor than in PD, and are accompanied by hallucinations (typically visual in nature and well-formed – in the memory clinic we hear about children playing in yards that no one else can see) and this is dementia due to Lewy bodies. The same Lewy bodies are seen in dementia with Lewy bodies as are seen in PD; however, in this disease, they are not mostly in the deep motor control areas of the brain but are there *and* in other areas responsible for cognitive function. Commonly, dementia with Lewy bodies is associated with slowing of the speed of mental processing, problems with complex attention, executive function problems, memory problems, and problems understanding one's visual and spatial world (Outeiro et al., 2019).

*Additional movement-based diseases.* Other causes of dementia that impact the motor system include dementia due to Huntington's disease, a disease characterized by excessive movements and cognitive, behavioural, and psychiatric changes. People can, however, live with Huntington's disease for years before being diagnosed with dementia (McColgan & Tabrizi, 2018). Progressive super nuclear palsy is a movement problem predominantly of eye gaze but progresses quickly and can be a cause of dementia (Golbe, 2014). Corticobasal degeneration can cause problems sequencing motor movements and additional cognitive problems consistent with dementia (Armstrong et al., 2014).

*Frontotemporal dementias.* Not long ago, one variant of frontotemporal dementia (FTD) was called Pick's disease. Our thinking on FTD has evolved to include many possible conditions (such as progressive supranuclear palsy or corticobasal degeneration), disorders that primarily impact language and disorders that primarily impact personality and behaviour. We used to think of these as distinct, but now understand that for many people they are linked – and some have common genetic components (Yokoyama et al., 2017). We are not entirely sure that we have discovered the type of cell death common to many of the variants of FTD, but progress is ongoing. FTD tends to be diagnosed at younger ages, most commonly in one's fifties, but there is a lot of variability in the age of onset (Bang et al., 2015). One variant of FTD impacts a person's personality and behaviour and this is sometimes referred to as the frontal or behavioural variant of FTD. Personality changes can be what looks like a lack of motivation but no sad mood, people might not speak much or not speak at all unless spoken to, and they have difficulties with reasoning or problem solving. A more common personality change presentation is people who act in socially inappropriate ways, do not appear to understand the feelings of others (but used to be highly empathetic), act impulsively, demonstrate poor judgement (which was a change for them), focus on engaging in pleasurable activities, which for some results in excessive eating of sweets or for others hypersexual behaviours (Bang et al., 2015). It can be hard to tell this apart from psychiatric conditions. People can be misdiagnosed with bipolar affective disorder due to the dramatic changes in personality, but if accompanied by motor changes (some features of parkinsonism are common) and problems progress over time, psychiatrists will refer to memory clinics or to dementia specialists for diagnosis. FTD is also characterized by two language variants – progressive non-fluent aphasia and semantic dementia (see below) (Bang et al., 2015). It can be confusing because sometimes these language variants are discussed along with FTD and sometimes they are referred to as progressive aphasias. Our thinking has evolved to include them in the FTD category because when people are diagnosed with these aphasias and their symptoms progress, they show more of the frontal and behavioural problems discussed above as characteristic of the frontal variant of FTD. Nevertheless, the symptoms are quite unique, so in this chapter we will discuss them separately.

---

Carmel notes her experience with her mother:

As Mum's diagnosis was received so late into her journey, we had no idea what was causing her out- of-character actions. Her personality was so immense; Mum had always been a quiet, practical, uncomplicated lady who loved her home and family. Mum became aggressive, using language I did not believe she even knew. She was so distracted; she would have spells of this out-of-character behaviour and then return to my beautiful, sweet mother. If we had been told about what the diagnosis would mean and do, we could have been prepared and not frightened of the episodes. Also Mum became nonverbal for her final year.

---

*Progressive aphasias.* Difficulties expressing oneself fluently, frequent mispronunciation of words, halting effortful speech, speech that is mostly nouns and verbs and is not grammatically correct, or general lack of speech are characteristic of progressive non-fluent aphasia or the non-fluent variant of FTD. Despite difficulties with expressing oneself, understanding others is relatively easy to do. This can look a lot like a common aphasia after a stroke – Broca's aphasia; however, in Broca's aphasia language gets better over time (or remains stable), and in non-fluent FTD, language problems worsen and begin to include other cognitive, motor, and behavioural changes. Another progressive aphasia called logogenic aphasia is similar in presentation to non-fluent aphasia in terms of symptoms, but it has the cell death of plaques and tangles that is typically seen in AD. Semantic dementia presents as someone who might have a hard time communicating because they can't recall the word for housecat, and might say tiger instead. Speech is lacking in nouns, and non-descriptive terms like 'that' or 'thing' might become more frequently used. Over time, the cell death impacts more of the networks in the brain where facts and definitions of words/objects are stored, and this impacts the ability to understand others or identify objects. As the disease progresses, more features of other variants of FTD are evident. Typically for progressive aphasias, function is relatively well-preserved in the early stages of the diseases, provided communication is not necessary for function (Bang et al., 2015).

*Head injuries and dementia.* Traumatic brain injuries vary from mild to severe, and have been linked to increased dementia risk. Mild traumatic brain injuries are sometimes referred to as concussions when paired with sports. There seems to be a specific type of cell death seen on autopsy for persons who commonly have a history of multiple traumatic brain injuries, and this has been labelled chronic traumatic encephalopathy (CTE). This is a controversial diagnosis made after death and, at the time of writing this book, is not a diagnosis used clinically – much more research is needed (Iverson et al., 2015). Moderate or severe traumatic brain injuries can leave people with multiple areas of cognitive impairment that also negatively impact their ability to function independently in daily life; however, they are not considered under the rubric of dementia, rather they are considered an acquired brain injury.

Another type of injury to the brain can cause multiple problems in cognition and function that might not necessarily be neurodegenerative; it is not considered under the rubric of dementias but is considered an acquired brain injury. For example, Wernicke–Korsakoff syndrome (WKS) is a disorder of the brain caused by a deficiency of vitamin B1 (thiamine) that is brought on by alcohol abuse in the context of nutritional deficiency (people who engage in an excessive intake of alcohol get their calories from alcohol and can have a very poor diet which leads to thiamine deficiency). In Ireland, those who present with WKS are unfortunately not getting a diagnosis or the supports they need (Alcohol Action Ireland, 2020). Many are falling through the cracks as they become unemployed, homeless, or are supported in nursing home facilities. Ireland, like many other countries, has a history of alcohol abuse, and while awareness campaigns have been successful there is still a major problem over all age brackets. Historically, it would have been the male population who were the main cohort; however, in recent years, the female population is being affected as well. Malnutrition can also result in Korsakoff syndrome. Many of our population for various reasons are living below the poverty line so a balanced nutritional diet is not being achieved (Arya, 1995).

## CAN I PREVENT DEMENTIA?

The thought that dementia can be prevented is relatively new, and there is vigorous research on modifiable risk factors for dementia; a whole chapter could be dedicated to this topic. Essentially, anything that is healthy for you – reducing conditions like high blood pressure, eating a diet high in healthy fats and proteins and low in processed foods, avoiding excessive alcohol intake, engaging in physical activity, paying attention to your mental health, which includes socializing with others – has been shown to reduce the risk of dementia. Acquiring formal education earlier in life and ensuring you remain mentally active – including maintaining your hearing acuity with hearing aids if needed and correcting your vision – have been shown to be modifiable risk factors for dementia (Baumgart et al., 2015; Livingston et al., 2020; Thomson et al., 2017).

To understand how dementia can be prevented, it is important to have an understanding of the relation between biological disease processes, referred to as pathologies, and their interaction with other variables that lead to nerve cell death or neurodegeneration. First, it is likely that many people who experience dementia probably have more than one pathological process impacting their brain (co-pathologies). Earlier in the chapter, we discussed the example of AD pathology interacting with vascular pathologies, which is a common co-pathology. Research into ways to measure pathologies in the brain of people who are experiencing dementia has exploded in recent years and will likely continue to help shape how we view dementia in the context of co-pathologies, and might even help us understand how these co-pathologies interact to increase the risk of dementia. The current state of the evidence on biomarkers of brain pathology hints that science has a lot more to understand about pathological processes in the brain and their relation to cognitive dysfunction and possible dementia. An example comes from subgroups of the American population and the pathologies of beta-amyloid and p-tau that are biomarkers of AD, which will be explained in more detail below.

The typically understood model of AD is that there is a buildup of beta-amyloid in the brain many years before the onset of any visible signs or symptoms of cognitive decline. Then, at some point, there is a buildup of p-tau in the brain. Neurodegeneration then becomes noticeable and when it is more extensive it is possible to clinically measure cognitive decline. At a certain threshold after which cognitive decline is sufficiently severe to impact a person's ability to function independently in daily life, a diagnosis of dementia is warranted. The beta-amyloid and p-tau continue to build up in the brain, causing further neurodegeneration and resulting in additional cognitive and functional decline. This biological model of AD or the amyloid-tau-neurodegeneration (ATN) framework (van der Flier & Scheltens, 2022) is well accepted, but science has also shown that not all people with AD show evidence of both beta-amyloid and p-tau. For example, some data suggest that African-American males with AD have biomarkers suggesting the presence of beta-amyloid in the absence of p-tau (Modeste et al., 2023). It is likely that co-pathologies interact with sex and ethnic background in different ways that future research needs to help explain.

How these brain pathologies develop and how they continue to build up is another topic of vigorous research. Some of the factors that contribute to the development of brain pathologies are inherited. Some of the inherited factors are genetic, based in the deoxyribonucleic acid (DNA), which is inherited. Some of these factors are based in DNA but are not directly inherited. Human cells divide repeatedly throughout the lifespan, and this can result in mutations in the DNA carried in each human cell (like base-pair deletions or substitutions), and some of these changes in DNA are common with ageing (such as shortening telomeres of the DNA-based chromosomes). DNA is important because it provides instructions for cells to produce intracellular proteins. The proteins in cells are how the cells do their job to live, replicate, keep themselves healthy, and die as needed. Protein expression within cells depends on genes in DNA (that creates a ribonucleic acid [RNA] 'recipe'), but protein expression also depends on additional factors. Factors that turn on or off protein expression are almost as important as the gene on the DNA that provides the recipe for creating the protein. Epigenetic factors are heritable, but these factors do not change the DNA; rather, they change the on/off switch for how proteins are expressed from genes on the DNA. Genetic (some genetic factors are inherited and some are a result of mutations) and epigenetic factors interact to increase or decrease the risk of dementia in ways that future research will help to explain (Maloney & Lahiri, 2016). Factors that turn on or off protein expression include those related to other aspects of biology that impact cells, such as general metabolic functions, hormones, and immune system function. Factors outside the human body can also impact how human cells function and help influence protein expression within cells. Some examples include exposure to diseases and toxins, and lifestyle factors such as nutritional health and physical activity and exercise. All these factors interact to increase or decrease the risk of dementia.

For many years, science detailed associations between lifestyle factors and the risk of dementia, and in 2020 the Lancet Commission (Livingston et al., 2020) helped to focus researchers and clinicians on modifiable risk factors for dementia. The Lancet Commission's careful review of the available scientific literature includes exposures to risk factors as dependent on life course – some risk factor exposures in, for example mid-life, impacted the risk of dementia in later life. The synthesis of the literature resulted in an estimate that 40% of dementias are related to modifiable risk factors. They detailed the following 12 risk factors that could be modifiable, and if modified could help prevent dementia: (1) in early life having access to education (literacy is particularly important); in midlife or sooner (2) treating hearing loss, (3) avoiding traumatic brain injury, (4) treating or avoiding high blood pressure, (5) reducing alcohol intake, (6) avoiding or addressing obesity; and in later life or sooner (7) avoiding or ceasing smoking cigarettes, (8) avoiding or treating depression, (9) avoiding or addressing social isolation, (10) avoiding or addressing physical inactivity, (11) avoiding or treating diabetes, and (12) avoiding air pollution.

The pioneering study called the Finnish Geriatric Intervention Study to Prevent Cognitive Impairment and Disability (FINGER) helped shift the focus of dementia research to include interventions for dementia prevention by researching a multicomponent intervention (Kivipelto et al., 2013). The FINGER (Kivipelto et al., 2013) and World-Wide FINGERS (Kivipelto et al., 2020) as well as the Fifth Canadian Consensus Conference on the Diagnosis and Treatment of Dementia (CCCDTD-5; Ismail et al., 2020) stressed the importance of targeting modifiable lifestyle factors across multiple domains. The original FINGER study demonstrated that those in the intervention group had better cognitive performance at two-year follow-up than those in the control group (Ngandu et al., 2015). The FINGER intervention (Kivipelto et al., 2013) included individualized nutritional advice focused on consuming a large amount of fruits and vegetables each day, eating fish at least twice a week, consuming low-fat milk and meats, reducing the amount of sugar consumed in a day, and swapping margarine for butter. A physical training programme was also individualized and progressive – it became increasingly more involved (at the end, it was 45–60 minutes three to five times a week) and included strength-based exercises and aerobic exercises. They also had ten group-based cognitive training sessions led by a psychologist, which was considered a cognitively stimulating and sociable activity, and was followed by independent training sessions three times a week on computers. Finally, frequent medical visits ensured that metabolic and vascular risk factors were treated on an individualized basis. Many other countries have begun similar prevention trials and additional follow-up evaluations have been conducted (see https://www.alz.org/research/for_researchers/grants/types-of -grants/alzheimers-association-world-wide-fingers-network for updated information as it becomes available).

The literature on prevention refers to reducing risk factors in the hope of delaying dementia onset. If dementia is delayed at the level of the population, people will die of other causes before dementia becomes apparent (Zissimopoulos et al., 2018). At the time of writing this book, there are no disease-modifying medications that can prevent dementia (Belder et al., 2023). Hopefully, this part of the book does not age well. Van der Flier et al. (2023) postulate that the future of personalized approaches that include medications to target different pathologies in the brain or influence protein expression together with lifestyle changes can lead to dementia prevention. Science first needs to understand all possible co-pathologies that cause dementia and develop medications that reduce these pathologies in the brain. Two medications targeting beta-amyloid were approved by the US Food and Drug Administration. One medication, Aducanumab, was approved in 2021 but has been discontinued as of 2024 so that the company can focus on Lecanemab, which was approved in 2023 and appears more promising. Lecanemab is being prescribed but its side-effect profile means close monitoring is required. (See https:// www.alz.org/alzheimers-dementia/treatments/medications-for -memory for up-to-date medication information.) We are hopeful that medications targeting a number of different pathological processes in the brain will be available in the coming years. In 2024, many medications for dementia that are in their final stage of medication development (Stage 3) are being studied. Most of these medications focus on modifying the pathological causes of dementia in the brain (some focus on amyloid and others on p-tau or other pathologies), and treatment with these medications will likely be tied to biomarker support for the presence of pathological processes in the brain. Other medications currently under study focus on enhancing cognition or addressing the behavioural and psychiatric symptoms of dementia (Cummings et al., 2024).

## IS THERE A WAY TO DELAY THE ONSET OF DEMENTIA?

The available research suggests that there might be a way to delay the onset of dementia, but much of what one needs to do is similar to what one needs to do to reduce the risk of dementia, which was discussed in the section on dementia prevention. Engage in a heart-healthy lifestyle, maintain cognitive and social activity, and manage diseases like diabetes, high blood pressure, and high cholesterol. Of the healthy behaviours to engage in, however, physical activity and exercise have been shown to be the most important factor in carefully controlled trials to maintain the volume of the brain region reasonable for memory and can delay the transition from mild cognitive impairment to dementia due to AD. The reasons for this are likely due to the interactions of multiple factors, but what is good for your heart health is good for your brain health. Many causes of dementia likely include an interaction of the health of the blood flow to all areas of the brain with some additional form of cell death, which we referred to as co-pathologies. Moderate-intensity (you can still talk but are breathing noticeably faster) exercise for 30 minutes five times a week has the most research support for potentially delaying dementia (Nelson et al., 2007), but the FINGERS study helps us see the benefit of a multicomponent intervention (Kivipelto et al., 2013) that includes not only physical activity and exercise but also diet modification, cognitive and social stimulation, and the management of metabolic and cardiovascular health.

# WHAT ARE THE GENETICS OF DEMENTIA?

Much of the response to this question depends on the disease underlying the dementia, and as you can tell from reading the above, multiple different diseases cause dementia, and these disease processes interact with a multitude of factors. Some of the genetic diseases have been clearly established: trisomy 21, which causes Down syndrome, will cause AD in people who have Down syndrome and live into their late thirties/early forties. Some other causes of AD are genetic, tending towards people who are diagnosed with AD in their fifties (also referred to as young onset dementia) – typically most people who are diagnosed with AD are well into their 80th decade or older. Some of the causes of frontotemporal dementias that tend to be diagnosed in the 60th decade have a clear genetic component, but many do not, likely because they have not yet been identified. Huntington's disease, which tends to present as a motor disease in the 60th decade, has a clear genetic component (Loy et al., 2014). Most cases of dementia likely result from causes that have a genetic and epigenetic component (Maloney & Lahiri, 2016) and likely interact with lifestyle factors to increase or decrease dementia risk.

# AM I MORE LIKELY TO GET DEMENTIA IF IT RUNS IN MY FAMILY?

How does one know if there is a clear genetic component without looking at the diseases tested for in 23andme? They look at the extended family and the history of diseases, which is why we ask about family history in one author's memory clinic. This is not always simple because AD diagnosed in one's seventies or later is so common that it looks like it runs in families. An easy way to remember this is that the later the age of onset of AD, the less likely it is to have a genetic component. People who have two copies of genes tied to AD (apo e-4), are more likely to be diagnosed with AD in their sixties, one copy a bit older in age, and for those with no copies, dementia due to AD can be diagnosed as well but tends to be later in the 80th and into the 90th decade of life. Despite knowing that apo e-4 is associated with an increased risk for AD, advanced age remains the larger predictive factor for most people, and this is why routine genetic testing is not done clinically for later age onset AD (Koriath et al., 2021). At the time of writing this book, most causes of dementia do not have a clear genetic component because genetic, epigenetic, and additional factors such as those that impact general health interact with pathologies in the brain to contribute to the risk of dementia (Maloney & Lahiri, 2016).

---

Carmel reflects on her learning from the diagnostic process:

No one is guaranteed what their future holds, but after witnessing my Mum's transformation over the ten years, I am in a better place to put tools in place to help myself have a better quality of later age life. I know the importance of a good diet, regular exercise, keeping my brain active and challenged.

Most importantly, I realize I must protect myself and remain connected to my community, not let myself become isolated or marginalized, it is so important to remain in contact with like-minded people and be kind to yourself. I also know the practical things to do, for example, to have my affairs in order, have my health directive in place, and my living will documented. We will be discussing such issues in subsequent chapters.

---

## CHAPTER 1 RESOURCES

These selected resources are a good place to start finding accessible guides. It is not an exhaustive list nor does it cover all countries and different legal jurisdictions.

Alzheimer Society. (n.d.-a). *Brain-healthy tips to reduce your risk of dementia.* Alzheimer Society of Canada. Retrieved March 31, 2024, from https://

alzheimer.ca/en/about-dementia/how-can-i-reduce-risk-dementia/brain-healthy-tips-reduce-your-risk-dementia

Alzheimer Society. (n.d.-b). *Managing the changes in your abilities*. Alzheimer Society of Canada. Retrieved March 31, 2024, from https://alzheimer.ca/en/help-support/im-living-dementia/managing-changes-your-abilities

Alzheimer Society. (2023). *Getting a diagnosis toolkit*. https://alzheimer.ca/sites/default/files/documents/getting-a-diagnosis-toolkit.pdf

Alzheimer's Association. (2021). *Dementia-related behaviors*. https://www.alz.org/media/documents/alzheimers-dementia-related-behaviors-ts.pdf

Alzheimer's Association. (2024a). Alzheimer's Association World Wide FINGERS Network Funding Program (ALZ WW-FNFP). https://www.alz.org/research/for_researchers/grants/types-of-grants/alzheimers-association-world-wide-fingers-network

Alzheimer's Association. (2024b). Medications for memory, cognition and dementia-related behaviors. https://www.alz.org/alzheimers-dementia/treatments/medications-for-memory

Alzheimer's Society. (2021). *Fact sheet genetics of dementia*. https://www.alzheimers.org.uk/sites/default/files/pdf/factsheet_genetics_of_dementia.pdf

Brennan, S. (2013, October 18). *I have trouble remembering things does that mean I am getting dementia?* https://vimeo.com/77213314

Dementia Australia. (n.d.). *Living with dementia*. Retrieved March 31, 2024, from https://www.dementia.org.au/living-dementia

Interior Health. (2018). *When your loved one has dementia*. https://divisionsbc.ca/sites/default/files/pedney/Dementia%20Booklet%20v23_FNL%20Aug_23_2018_electronic.pdf

Logan, B., & M.S.W. (n.d.). *Caregiver's guide to understanding dementia behaviors*. Family Caregiver Alliance. Retrieved March 31, 2024, from https://www.caregiver.org/resource/caregivers-guide-understanding-dementia-behaviors/

# REFERENCES

Abrams, L., & Davis, D. (2016). The tip-of-the-tongue phenomenon. In H. H. Wright (Ed.), *Cognition, language, and aging* (pp. 13–53). John Benjamins Publishing Company. https://doi.org/10.1075/z.200.02abr

Alcohol Action Ireland. (2020, December 8). Ireland's first ever seminar on Korsakoff's Syndrome. *Alcohol Action Ireland*. https://alcoholireland.ie/irelands-first-ever-seminar-korsakoffs-syndrome/

Allain, P., Etcharry-Bouyx, F., & Verny, C. (2013). Executive functions in clinical and preclinical Alzheimer's disease. *Revue Neurologique, 169*(10), 695–708. https://doi.org/10.1016/j.neurol.2013.07.020

American Psychiatric Association. (2022). *Diagnostic and statistical manual of mental disorders* (5th ed.) (pp. 509–596). https://doi.org/10.1176/appi.books.9780890425787

Armstrong, M. J. (2014). Diagnosis and treatment of corticobasal degeneration. *Current Treatment Options in Neurology, 16,* 1–12. https://doi.org/10.1007/s11940-013-0282-1

Arya, D. K. (1995). Wernicke-Korsakoff syndrome following self-induced starvation. *Irish Journal of Psychological Medicine, 12*(2), 66–67. https://doi.org/10.1017/S0790966700004249

Bang, J., Spina, S., & Miller, B. L. (2015). Frontotemporal dementia. *The Lancet, 386*(10004), 1672–1682. https://doi.org/10.1016/S0140-6736(15)00461-4

Baumgart, M., Snyder, H. M., Carrillo, M. C., Fazio, S., Kim, H., & Johns, H. (2015). Summary of the evidence on modifiable risk factors for cognitive decline and dementia: A population-based perspective. *Alzheimer's & Dementia, 11*(6), 718–726. https://doi.org/10.1016/j.jalz.2015.05.016

Belder, C. R., Schott, J. M., & Fox, N. C. (2023). Preparing for disease-modifying therapies in Alzheimer's disease. *The Lancet Neurology, 22*(9), 782–783. https://doi.org/10.1016/S1474-4422(23)00274-0

Cummings J, Zhou Y, Lee G, Zhong K, Fonseca J, Cheng F. (2024). Alzheimer's disease drug development pipeline: 2024. *Alzheimers Dement (New York, N. Y.).* 10(2):e12465. doi: 10.1002/trc2.12465.

El Haj, M., Colombel, F., Kapogiannis, D., & Gallouj, K. (2020). False memory in Alzheimer's disease. *Behavioural Neurology, 2020,* 5284504. https://doi.org/10.1155/2020/5284504

Franzen, S., van den Berg, E., Goudsmit, M., Jurgens, C. K., van de Wiel, L., Kalkisim, Y., Uysal-Bozkir, Ö., Ayhan, Y., Nielsen, T. R., & Papma, J. M. (2020). A systematic review of neuropsychological tests for the assessment of dementia in non-Western, low-educated or illiterate populations. *Journal of the International Neuropsychological Society, 26*(3), 331–351. https://doi.org/10.1017/S1355617719000894

Goncalves, J. T., Schafer, S. T., & Gage, F. H. (2016). Adult neurogenesis in the hippocampus: From stem cells to behavior. *Cell, 167*(4), 897–914. https://doi.org/10.1016/j.cell.2016.10.021

Golbe L. I. (2014). Progressive supranuclear palsy. *Seminars in Neurology, 34*(2), 151–159. https://doi.org/10.1055/s-0034-1381736

Health Service Executive. (2023). Public health nurses and community registered general nurses (Onmsd). https://healthservice.hse.ie/about-us/onmsd/onmsd/specific-programmes/phn-community-registered-general-nurses.html

Ismail, Z., Black, S. E., Camicioli, R., Chertkow, H., Herrmann, N., Laforce, R., Jr, Montero-Odasso, M., Rockwood, K., Rosa-Neto, P.,

Seitz, D., Sivananthan, S., Smith, E. E., Soucy, J. P., Vedel, I., Gauthier, S., & CCCDTD5 participants (2020). Recommendations of the 5th Canadian Consensus Conference on the diagnosis and treatment of dementia. *Alzheimer's & Dementia: The Journal of the Alzheimer's Association, 16*(8), 1182–1195. https://doi.org/10.1002/alz.12105

Iverson, G. L., Gardner, A. J., McCrory, P., Zafonte, R., & Castellani, R. J. (2015). A critical review of chronic traumatic encephalopathy. *Neuroscience & Biobehavioral Reviews, 56,* 276–293. doi: 10.1016/j.neubiorev.2015.05.008

Jack, C. R. Jr, Bennett, D. A., Blennow, K., Carrillo, M. C., Dunn, B., Haeberlein, S. B., Holtzman, D. M., Jagust, W., Jessen, F., Karlawish, J., Liu, E., Molinuevo, J. L., Montine, T., Phelps, C., Rankin, K. P., Rowe, C. C., Scheltens, P., Siemers, E., Snyder, H. M., ... & Sperling R (2018). NIA-AA research framework: Toward a biological definition of Alzheimer's disease. *Alzheimer's & Dementia, 14*(4), 535–562. https://doi: 10.1016/j.jalz.2018.02.018

Kivipelto, M., Mangialasche, F., Snyder, H. M., Allegri, R., Andrieu, S., Arai, H., Baker, L., Belleville, S., Brodaty, H., Brucki, S. M., Calandri, I., Caramelli, P., Chen, C., Chertkow, H., Chew, E., Choi, S. H., Chowdhary, N., Crivelli, L., De La Torre, R., ... & Carrillo, M. C. (2020). World-Wide FINGERS Network: A global approach to risk reduction and prevention of dementia. *Alzheimer's & dementia, 16*(7), 1078–1094. https://doi.org/10.1002/alz.12123

Kivipelto, M., Solomon, A., Ahtiluoto, S., Ngandu, T., Lehtisalo, J., Antikainen, R., Bäckman, L., Hänninen, T., Jula, A., Laatikainen, T., Lindström, J., Mangialasche, F., Nissinen, A., Paajanen, T., Pajala, S., Peltonen, M., Rauramaa, R., Stigsdotter-Neely, A., Strandberg, T., ... & Soininen, H. (2013). The Finnish geriatric intervention study to prevent cognitive impairment and disability (FINGER): Study design and progress. *Alzheimer's & Dementia, 9*(6), 657–665. https://doi.org/10.1016/j.jalz.2012.09.012

Korczyn A. D. (2002). Mixed dementia--the most common cause of dementia. *Annals of the New York Academy of Sciences, 977,* 129–134. https://doi.org/10.1111/j.1749-6632.2002.tb04807.x

Koriath, C. A., Kenny, J., Ryan, N. S., Rohrer, J. D., Schott, J. M., Houlden, H., Fox, N. C., Tabrizi, S. J., & Mead, S. (2021). Genetic testing in dementia—utility and clinical strategies. *Nature Reviews Neurology, 17*(1), 23–36. https://doi.org/10.1038/s41582-020-00416-1

Kumari, N. (2023, October 11). Sligo woman's courageous battle for the rights of those with dementia. *Irish Independent.* https://www.independent.ie/regionals/sligo/news/sligo-womans-courageous-battle-for-the-rights-of-those-with-dementia/a570679009.html

Lethbridge, L., Johnston, G. M., & Turnbull, G. (2013). Co-morbidities of persons dying of Parkinson's disease. *Progress in Palliative Care, 21*(3), 140–145. https://doi.org/10.1179/1743291X12Y.0000000037

Livingston, G., Huntley, J., Sommerlad, A., Ames, D., Ballard, C., Banerjee, S., Brayne, C., Burns, A., Cohen-Mansfield, J., Cooper, C., Costafreda, S. G., Dias, A., Fox, N., Gitlin, L. N., Howard, R., Kales, H. C., Kivimäki, M., Larson, E. B., Ogunniyi, A.,... & Mukadam, N. (2020). Dementia prevention, intervention, and care: 2020 report of the Lancet Commission. *The Lancet, 396*(10248), 413–446. https://doi.org/10.1016/S0140-6736(20)30367-6

Loy, C. T., Schofield, P. R., Turner, A. M., & Kwok, J. B. (2014). Genetics of dementia. *The Lancet, 383*(9919), 828–840. https://doi.org/10.1016/S0140-6736(13)60630-3

Maloney, B., & Lahiri, D. K. (2016). Epigenetics of dementia: Understanding the disease as a transformation rather than a state. *The Lancet Neurology, 15*(7), 760–774.

Mattison, M. L. P. (2020). Delirium. *Annals of Internal Medicine, 173*(7), 509–596. https://doi.org/10.7326/AITC202010060

McColgan, P., & Tabrizi, S. J. (2018). Huntington's disease: A clinical review. *European Journal of Neurology, 25*(1), 24–34. https://doi.org/10.1111/ene.13413

Modeste, E. S., Ping, L., Watson, C. M., Duong, D. M., Dammer, E. B., Johnson, E. C. B., Roberts, B. R., Lah, J. J., Levey, A. I., & Seyfried, N. T. (2023). Quantitative proteomics of cerebrospinal fluid from African Americans and Caucasians reveals shared and divergent changes in Alzheimer's disease. *Molecular Neurodegeneration, 18,* 48. https://doi.org/10.1186/s13024-023-00638-z

Morgan, D. G., Walls-Ingram, S., Cammer, A., O'Connell, M. E., Crossley, M., Dal Bello-Haas, V., Forbes, D., Innes, A., Kirk, A., & Stewart, N. (2014). Informal caregivers' hopes and expectations of a referral to a memory clinic. *Social Science & Medicine, 102,* 111–118. https://doi.org/10.1016/j.socscimed.2013.11.023

Nelson, M. E., Rejeski, W. J., Blair, S. N., Duncan, P. W., Judge, J. O., King, A. C., Macera, C. A., & Castaneda-Sceppa, C. (2007). Physical activity and public health in older adults: Recommendation from the American College of Sports Medicine and the American Heart Association. *Circulation, 116*(9), 1094. https://www.doi.org/10.1161/CIRCULATIONAHA.107.185650

Ngandu, T., Lehtisalo, J., Solomon, A., Levälahti, E., Ahtiluoto, S., Antikainen, R., Bäckman, L., Hänninen, T., Jula, A., Laatikainen, T., Lindström, J., Mangialasche, F., Paajanen, T., Pajala, S., Markku Peltonen, M., Rauramaa, R., Stigsdotter-Neely, A., Strandberg, T., Tuomilehto, J., ... & Kivipelto, M. (2015). A 2 year multidomain intervention of diet, exercise, cognitive training, and vascular risk monitoring versus control to prevent cognitive decline in at-risk elderly people (FINGER): A randomised controlled trial. *The Lancet, 385*(9984), 2255–2263. https://doi.org/10.1016/S0140-6736(15)60461-5

Nobis, L., & Husain, M. (2018). Apathy in Alzheimer's disease. *Current Opinion in Behavioral Sciences, 22*, 7–13. https://doi.org/10.1016/j.cobeha.2017.12.007

O'Connell, M. E., Crossley, M., Cammer, A., Morgan, D., Allingham, W.★, Cheavins, B.★, Dalziel, D.★, Lemire, M.★, Mitchell, S.★, & Morgan, E.★ (2014). Development and evaluation of a telehealth videoconferenced support group for rural spouses of individuals diagnosed with atypical early-onset dementias. *Dementia: The International Journal of Social Research and Practice, 13*(3), 382–395. https://doi.org/10.1177/1471301212474143 ★caregiver participant collaborators.

O'Connell, M. E., Kadlec, H., Maimon, G., Taler, V., Simard, M., Griffith, L., Tuokko, H., Voll, S., Wolfson, C., Kirkland, S., & Raina, P. (2021). Methodological considerations when establishing reliable and valid normative data: Canadian Longitudinal Study on Aging (CLSA) neuropsychological battery. *The Clinical Neuropsychologist, 36*(8), 2168–2187. https://doi.org/10.1080/13854046.2021.1954243

Outeiro, T. F., Koss, D. J., Erskine, D., Walker, L., Kurzawa-Akanbi, M., Burn, D., Donaghy, P., Morris, C., Taylor, J-P., Thomas, A., Attems, J., & McKeith, I. (2019). Dementia with Lewy bodies: An update and outlook. *Molecular Neurodegeneration, 14*, 1–18. https://doi.org/10.1186/s13024-019-0306-8

Overman, M. J., Leeworthy, S., & Welsh, T. J. (2021). Estimating premorbid intelligence in people living with dementia: A systematic review. *International Psychogeriatrics, 33*(11), 1145–1159. https://doi.org/10.1017/S1041610221000302

Ruggiero, C., Baroni, M., Xenos, D., Parretti, L., Macchione, I. G., Bubba, V., Laudisio, A., Pedone, C., Ferracci, M., Magierski, R., Boccardi, V., Antonelli-Incalzi, R., & Mecocci, P. (2024). Dementia, osteoporosis and fragility fractures: Intricate epidemiological relationships, plausible biological connections, and twisted clinical practices. *Ageing Research Reviews, 93*, 102130. https://doi.org/10.1016/j.arr.2023.102130

Salthouse, T. A. (2010). Selective review of cognitive aging. *Journal of the International Neuropsychological Society, 16*(5), 754–760. https://doi.org/10.1017/S1355617710000706

Salthouse, T. A. (2016). *Theoretical perspectives on cognitive aging.* Psychology Press.

Teunissen, C. E., Verberk, I. M. W., Thijssen, E. H., Vermunt, L., Hansson, O., Zetterberg, H., van der Flier, W. M., Mielke, M. M., & Del Campo, M. (2022). Blood-based biomarkers for Alzheimer's disease: Towards clinical implementation. *The Lancet Neurology, 21*(1), 66–77. https://doi.org /10.1016/S1474-4422(21)00361-6

Thomson, R. S., Auduong, P., Miller, A. T., & Gurgel, R. K. (2017). Hearing loss as a risk factor for dementia: A systematic review. *Laryngoscope Investigative Otolaryngology, 2*(2), 69–79. https://doi.org/10.1002/lio2.65

Todd, S., Barr, S., & Passmore, A. P. (2013). Cause of death in Alzheimer's disease: A cohort study. *QJM: Monthly Journal of the Association of Physicians, 106*(8), 747–753. https://doi.org/10.1093/qjmed/hct103

van der Flier, W. M., & Scheltens, P. (2022). The ATN Framework—Moving Preclinical Alzheimer disease to clinical relevance. *JAMA Neurology, 79*(10). 968–970. https://doi:10.1001/jamaneurol.2022.2967

van der Flier, W. M., de Vugt, M. E., Smets, E. M. A., Blom, M., & Teunissen, C. E. (2023). Towards a future where Alzheimer's disease pathology is stopped before the onset of dementia. *Nature Aging, 3*(5), 494–505. https:// doi: 10.1038/s43587-023-00404-2

Worthy, D. A., Gorlick, M. A., Pacheco, J. L., Schnyer, D. M., & Maddox, W. T. (2011). With age comes wisdom: Decision-making in younger and older adults. *Psychological Science, 22*(11), 1375–1380. https://doi.org/10 .1177/0956797611418471

Yokoyama, J. S., Karch, C. M., Fan, C. C., Bonham, L. W., Kouri, N., Ross, O. A., Rademakers, R., Kim, J., Wang, Y., Höglinger, G. U., Müller, U., Ferrari, R., Hardy, J., International FTD-Genomics Consortium (IFGC), Momeni, P., Sugrue, L. P., Hess, C. P., James Barkovich, A., Boxer, A. L., Seeley, W. W., … & Desikan, R. S. (2017). Shared genetic risk between corticobasal degeneration, progressive supranuclear palsy, and frontotemporal dementia. *Acta Neuropathologica, 133*(5), 825–837. https:// doi.org/10.1007/s00401-017-1693-y

Zissimopoulos, J. M., Tysinger, B. C., St. Clair, P. A., & Crimmins, E. M. (2018). The impact of changes in population health and mortality on future prevalence of Alzheimer's disease and other dementias in the United States. *The Journals of Gerontology: Series B, 73*(suppl_1), S38–S47. https:// doi.org/10.1093/geronb/gbx147

# 2

## HOW DO WE ADJUST TO
## LIFE WITH THE DIAGNOSIS?

### WHY DID I GET DEMENTIA?

Chapter 1 demonstrates that multiple disease processes underpin or cause dementia, and many of these diseases interact with other factors such as cardiovascular and cerebrovascular health, other health conditions, and cognitive reserve to increase or decrease the risk of dementia. Cognitive reserve refers to a construct first described when researchers were attempting to explain the gap between brain cell death and clinical dementia; some people in the study had substantial brain cell death usually associated with Alzheimer's disease; however, in their daily life before they passed away, they had no clinical signs of cognitive impairment or problems functioning independently (Snowden, 2003). The concept of cognitive reserve was explained to account for brains that could handle a very high degree of cell death due to Alzheimer's disease without it impacting cognition or function (Snowden, 2003; Stern, 2002). Some of an individual's cognitive reserve is related to years of formal education, how cognitively demanding a person's occupation was, how frequently do people engage in social activities or other cognitively demanding tasks, health variables including any health factors that impact the brain, and genetic luck. Some aspects of cognitive reserve are thought to be structural – more connections

DOI: 10.4324/9781003457138-3

in the brain due to education or cognitively stimulating activities – and some are thought to relate to how well a person can cognitively compensate for damaged circuits in the brain (Stern, 2002).

Although lifestyle factors can reduce dementia risk (Livingston et al., 2020) or increase cognitive reserve (Song et al., 2022), few would describe lifestyle factors alone as leading to or causing dementia. The closest possible example is vascular dementia that occurs due to repeated strokes. The risk of strokes is highly related to lifestyle factors that impact brain and heart health. However, it is not that simple; two people can have the same lifestyles but not have the same lifestyle-related diseases – multiple facets of genetic luck (e.g. genes for one's sex, genes for lipid levels, genes for diabetes mellitus) interact with lifestyle factors. In the end, there are things that people do that may increase or decrease their risk, but lifestyle factors on their own do not cause vascular dementia – it is a combination of factors that includes bad luck. Other underpinning risk factors, or causes of dementia, have an even more complicated relationship with lifestyle factors and, in the end, getting dementia is related to chance.

## WILL RECOVERY BE POSSIBLE?

Many people who are diagnosed with dementia may start to wonder if they can get better, if they can recover from this condition, or recover enough to be able to continue with their daily lives. Some people may self-impose the stigma that surrounds this condition. They may choose to hide the diagnosis from friends and family, or they may retreat into their own world. Their social circle may become smaller as fear of others finding out influences choices to continue to try to maintain social connections. It is at this point that a person may become depressed, not know where to turn for help, and choose to move forward alone. The person may choose not to tell other family members, who then may not know what's happening. People can be reluctant to disclose their diagnosis as they are worried about what it means for their lives or because they may believe that dementia is a mental health problem, and fear others' reactions. Or, some people may allow their loved ones to take over for them, as it is simpler than having to make decisions. Family members may feel compelled to make decisions, depending on how the diagnosis was given to them, who gave them the diagnosis and the words that were used, what information was offered to help support the person and their family, and what follow-up was planned.

Carmel's family experience demonstrates the difficulty of staying connected and recovering everyday life choices and preferences prior to being diagnosed.

Carmel reflects: 'Staying connected was difficult as friends and the community started to distance themselves. Now I know this was because, like us they did not understand what the diagnosis meant. Everyone was afraid – at times it felt like we were being isolated and punished. When neighbours visited, they spoke about Mum in the present tense and did not address her directly. This was so distressing for Mum and myself – trying to explain to them that Mum could hear them and understand them did not seem to register'.

The 'recovery' or adjustment phase of learning to live with the diagnosis and to understand what this means depends, in part, on the form or underlying cause of the dementia diagnosed, or the area of the brain affected. This is partially why no two journeys with dementia are alike. It is highly important for everyone to know the type of dementia and the possible causes, as this will help with understanding what is happening and finding ways to adjust and recover everyday life choices.

One of the first things anyone can advise a person living with dementia and their family is to give themselves the time to understand what is happening and to start to work out how to 'get your feet back under yourself'. Self-care is highly important at this point. Take the time needed to get life back on track. Talking with one's spouse and other trusted family members may help, as will speaking with the family doctor or a counsellor.

Counselling can be offered by a private counsellor, or charitable organizations such as the local Alzheimer Society office can also help, as they have people who know about dementia and who can provide information and education that may be of help. The Alzheimer Society and other similar organizations can direct either the person with the diagnosis or their family members to useful resources that suit individual circumstances. It is common that the person living with dementia (and their family) may feel like they are losing control of many aspects of daily life. This may include feelings of losing oneself, the person you have always been, and the person you have planned on being as you age. The person may question who they are and who they will become. This type of loss is known as loss of self (Sabat & Harre, 2008).

As Carmel reflects:

I didn't take time for self-care as I didn't have time to realize what was happening. One day runs into the next, and you are constantly playing catch up. Instead, I returned to education to arm myself with the knowledge and confidence I needed to be Mum's voice. I continued this after Mum's passing, which I found was a form of grieving. I am still advocating for the voice of our most vulnerable and campaigning daily for change in our health system.

Phyllis reflects on the different reactions of her closest family members:

Once the diagnosis was received, it seemed everyone had a different reaction or view on it. I personally was in shock but wanted to face it head on, deal with it, and move forward. My husband went into a state of denial; he could see nothing wrong. Each of the kids had their own thoughts on how to handle it. They ranged from ignoring it to taking over. It was at this point that I decided that I had to do what was right and felt comfortable for me. I needed to understand more, get educated, and take charge of myself. Others could assist me, but there was no way I was letting them take over. They needed to get educated on this also.

## HOW CAN I HELP SUPPORT SOMEONE LIVING WITH DEMENTIA?

Now what? This can be the question that anyone receiving the diagnosis and anyone in a support role may ask themselves. The diagnosis may lead to a state of disbelief. There can be many questions and no answers. After a diagnosis is given, perhaps there are medications to take, but often there may not have been any instructions as to what to do next. The person and their family may not even truly understand anything about the condition they have been diagnosed with. Some people may have some knowledge of dementia heard from others over time or know of a friend or a distant family member who had dementia or supported someone with dementia. At this time, many people living with dementia may feel the need, or indeed actually begin, to withdraw from everyday life; they may believe that their life is over as they knew it. The partner, family member, or friend of someone who has just received the diagnosis may well have similar questions to the person living with dementia, or they may be different. Family members may worry about how they will cope, how they can provide support, how they can learn more about the condition, and what they need to prepare themselves to take on in the way of support and care roles. But the diagnosis can also open doors for both the person diagnosed and their family members, doors to advice and support, doors to understanding that what is going on has a name, that there is an underlying reason for the issues that were causing concern.

As Carmel demonstrates while reflecting on her personal experience of her mother's diagnosis:

The diagnosis came as a relief; we now had a name for Mum's change of personality. We didn't get an explanation nor were we signposted to supports and services that we might need, but we left the neurologist feeling elated. Unfortunately, this was short-lived as we continued to struggle with day-to-day life without knowing and understanding what we were dealing with or what lay ahead. Looking back, if at the point of diagnosis a case worker had been assigned to Mum who would have directed us on the paths we needed to follow, life would have been so much easier. Lack of information was the biggest problem; the time and energy wasted on seeking help was not acceptable.

This highlights the need for support to be available to the family members and the person living with dementia as they begin to work out answers to the 'what next?' questions.

The person with the diagnosis and their family may begin to realize that there are going to be many other losses – loss of either the person with dementia or the family care partner's job, either because the person with dementia can no longer work in their role or they require increasing support that the care partner cannot provide if they continue their employment. There may be an associated loss of income when a wage earner is unable to continue to work. Some people will experience the loss of relationships or roles they held within their family and friendship groups. These losses can seem insurmountable, especially in the initial period of adjustment.

The personal reflections of Phyllis provide an indication of the losses that a person living with dementia may need support to adjust to following a diagnosis:

I will say this from personal experience. The first is the loss of who you are as a person and the loss of some of the abilities that you have. As an example, I worked as a nurse, which I felt I could no longer do after the diagnosis. I had to deal with, if I am no longer a nurse, who am I? and what can I do? Along with this came making decisions about leaving my job. If you're fortunate enough not to have lost your job due to mistakes you've made, I think you're better off because you go on your short-term disability and potentially your long-term disability, which does help financially. But if you've been fired already, you've lost your income, you've lost your work related benefits package, and these are all highly important to make sure you keep because it will make a difference in the long run. I had to deal with some of the complications I was having due to the disease process, such as no longer being able to fully read or comprehend what I was reading, and the loss of being able to do things on my own. A lot of times after this diagnosis, they require you to bring people with you to every appointment, so you lose your independence. It's at this time you may also lose your driver's license. It is at this point you feel like you've been hit in the gut and you've got nothing to go on for, and because you may not be thinking clearly due to the disease process, you may be having a hard time processing what's happening to you. It is also at this time that you may find you lose friends or family members. They may just quietly disappear from your life. You may not notice at first, but this happens. It may not be due to anything you have done; sometimes it's due to their lack of understanding of what is happening to you, their discomfort with the disease, or their own experiences with dementia. These things happen at a time when you are trying to adjust to a new way of life and are feeling overwhelmed. This is when you may either withdraw more or reach out for assistance from others, i.e. a counsellor or the Alzheimer Society. I would like to take a moment to reassure anyone supporting a person recently diagnosed, or the person with the diagnosis if you are reading this, that these are all just a part of the process you must go through to move on. It is at this time that you may become depressed due to the new situation that you find yourself in, but remember that it's okay to ask for help. You may even need medication to help you through as you come to terms with the diagnosis and adjust to what this might mean for your life.

Another important area where the person living with dementia may require support relates to nutrition and hydration. When living with dementia, eating well and remaining hydrated are important. It is too easy not to drink enough water, which really helps to keep us sharp and functioning well. We often don't take into consideration how important what we eat is; we eat what we want when we want it, and do not consider the nutritional value. Our bodies require nutrients and vitamins to function properly. The person may not feel like eating; this may be due to depression, complications of medication, or for reasons that are unknown. If this happens, or family become concerned about how the person with dementia is eating, it is important to seek advice and see someone about this (i.e. family doctor, nutritionist, counsellor). Daily nutritional requirements need to be considered to avoid causing other problems medically and to ensure that the physical body is receiving what it needs to function normally.

As Carmel reflects based on her experiences with her mother:

Eating advice is great, but the nutritionist or anyone else never mentioned the effect the diagnosis may have on the senses. When I discovered this, I started spicing up Mum's food; the results were amazing. I now realize the impact the disease was having on the various senses. Mum had been complaining about her hearing for a number of years, but nothing was done about it. One-on-one, Mum was able to follow and contribute, but now looking back, it was when there were more voices that she could not follow. Unfortunately, no clinician picked up on this, so the earliest symptom was missed.

A resource that Carmel found very helpful is *Talking Sense: Living with Sensory Changes and Dementia* – HammondCare Dementia Support (demsupport.org).

The physical signs or symptoms may be hindering the person's ability to meet their nutritional needs. Maybe there is 'brain fog', when the person simply forgets to eat or thinks they have already eaten. Medications may repress appetite. Or the brain may not be processing things properly. There may also be physical reasons such as swallowing problems, choking, tremors, or not knowing what one feels like eating. Many people notice that things previously enjoyed are no longer appetizing; taste buds may seem to have changed because the sense of smell commonly changes with many diseases that cause dementia (Barresi et al., 2012).

The following account from Phyllis exemplifies the multiple challenges she faced relating to food preparation and eating that came with her dementia:

Don't be alarmed by no longer liking the foods you enjoyed before; this can also happen due to the changes happening in your brain. My husband frequently teases me about not knowing what I eat anymore. What I want to eat and what I enjoy today may not necessarily be the same tomorrow. You may also find that making up your mind on what you want to eat becomes more difficult. Your ability to actually make the food may decline, and you may need assistance to do this.

I have always loved to cook, but I find it very difficult to do now. What I have come to realize is that I still love to cook, but I avoid doing it. My dementia has affected my ability to multitask, and when you are cooking, you are frequently multitasking. You are trying to prep and cook multiple dishes at the same time. As an example, if I am working on mashing potatoes while frying meat at the same time, I frequently burn the meat because I can only see the task I am working on, mashing the potatoes. So now, I may cook things in an order that allows me to make one thing at a time and reheat things later. The other thing we do in our house is that my husband has stepped in to help. He does this in two ways. On my good days, he will sit in the kitchen while I'm cooking, reading or playing a game, and he gives me gentle reminders as I go. The other way he assists is by doing most of the preparation and asking me for assistance. I will admit that it took me a while to accept the assistance, but now I actually love it as it allows me to still be able to participate in life. I may have to do things differently, but I can still do them.

The one thing I can definitely let you know is that accepting the changes that happen is not easy to do. You feel like you are losing your independence, but once you accept them, you can still live life to its fullest. You will have good days and bad days, but once you realize that this is okay, you will be able to move forward. Accept the help that is offered to you; it does help. The biggest thing for me was to change my way of thinking from I can't do this anymore, to look I can still do this. Take the negative reactions and turmoil and make them a positive. This gives you a feeling of I can still do things. Be open to accepting help when it is offered. I will also say that it is important to set limits and not let others take over for you. It may be easier for people who care about you to do this, and we may feel like it is easier for you, but it is important that we be able to still do things for ourselves. It gives us purpose and a feeling of accomplishment. You still have a lot of living to do; however, it may have to be done differently.

It is important to make plans and plan ahead. This helps you through things that you may find difficult and makes it easier for your family to assist. As an example, I used to have big family dinners on Sunday and everyone would come home. I can no longer organize and prepare these gatherings, so we have smaller gatherings. The larger gatherings are now done by my children at their homes. I can still participate by bringing a dish of food rather than stressing over making a full meal. I can find these gatherings overwhelming due to the noise, and I can feel like my brain is being overstimulated. As a family, we have found ways for me to still be part of this. For the noise, I wear noise-cancelling earbuds, and we have also set up a quiet area where I can retreat to calm down and rest my brain. We have also set up an exit plan, which means we may not be able to stay as long as we used to, but at least we were there. The other thing we do is monitor signs that I'm not doing well, like becoming very quiet and not participating; when this happens, my family intervenes by removing me to a different area or leaving the gathering entirely. We also prepare before we go by making sure I am dressed comfortably and am well-rested, which means I frequently take a nap before going to these events.

Some of the other things we have planned are for my future care. My wants and wishes are laid out, so others know and can implement them when necessary.

An important point to think about in relation to staying engaged is retaining a sense of purpose, value, and worth in day-to-day life. It is highly important that there are opportunities for the person living with dementia to stay engaged and social (Ward et al., 2022) to enable personal challenges to be set and met because by staying engaged and social, we can delay or slow the progression of dementia (Baumgart et al., 2015). This is discussed in more detail in Chapter 4. At this point, it is important to ensure that the person living with dementia is still able to, and encouraged to, participate in things that will, in turn, help to achieve a sense of purpose. There are a number of ways that the person living with dementia can retain purpose. One is by being an advocate, using one's voice to help change things not just for their own benefit but also for others living with dementia. When the person living with dementia tells their story, this can be a very powerful message and can help in the process of advocating for change and help to rewrite the perceptions and negative stories that often surround dementia. Living well with dementia and continuing to participate in social life can help change how people see dementia and change the stigma related to this disease. This can be a challenging thought for many; they think about how to protect the person living with dementia, and the person living with dementia may not want to be a burden or create any problems for their family. But there are many inspirational accounts of how those living with dementia can influence change. Take, for example, the 'Faces of Dementia' campaign that Phyllis was involved in.

Phyllis reflects on the benefits of her decision to stay involved:

Very soon after my diagnosis, I made the decision to stay involved and to try to make change to help those living with dementia, including myself and others. The Hamilton Council on Aging was successful in obtaining a Public Health Agency of Canada research grant to compare and implement a dementia-friendly community project, where they hoped to compare how a rural community and a city community might become dementia friendly. In doing this research, we also decided to do an anti-stigma campaign called the Faces of Dementia (www.facesofdementia.ca). This campaign focused on individuals living with dementia and staying involved in the community so that others can see that we are still us, and can still have a purpose. Being involved in this was truly life-changing for me as I felt engaged, I was able to be involved, and I had a purpose. I know I was not the only person in the campaign to feel this way. I have included the link above; please check it out and hear from others in the campaign – it may help you better understand people living with dementia.

There are many different groups out there for family members, for the person living with dementia, and for family members and people living with dementia to attend together. These include advocacy groups, support groups, and local advisory groups. It may be that the person living with dementia and/or their family can participate in research. Research is completely voluntary, and the person can join in as much or as little as they like. Some projects may sound fun, others interesting, and others may appear to offer hope for a cure or medication to help delay symptoms. Looking out for research opportunities is a good way to maintain connection and purpose.

As Phyllis argues from the perspective of someone living with dementia:

This is still your life, and you can still live it the way you want. I believe in the saying, if you don't use it, you lose it. Try to stay engaged and active as long as you can and enjoy life along the way. We still have living to do.

The challenge can be for others to find ways to enable the person living with dementia to continue to live their life on their terms, in ways that avoid exacerbating symptoms while still planning for the future. It is to the issue of future planning that we turn in Chapter 3.

## CHAPTER 2 RESOURCES

These selected resources are a good place to start to find accessible guides. It is not an exhaustive list, nor does it cover all countries and different legal jurisdictions.

Alzheimer Society. (2015a). *First steps for families.* https://alzheimer.ca/bc/sites/bc/files/documents/first_steps_for_families.pdf

Alzheimer Society. (2015b). *Ways to help.* https://alzheimer.ca/bc/sites/bc/files/documents/ways_to_help.pdf

Alzheimer Society. (2018). *COMMUNICATION.* https://alzheimer.ca/bc/sites/bc/files/documents/communication-2018.pdf

Alzheimer Society. (2019). *AMBIGUOUS LOSS AND GRIEF IN DEMENTIA.* https://alzheimer.ca/bc/sites/bc/files/documents/ambiguous-loss-and-grief_for-individuals-and-families.pdf

Alzheimer Society. (2022). *Progression overview* . https://alzheimer.ca/sites/default/files/documents/Progression-Overview-Alzheimer-Society.pdf

Alzheimer's Society. (2021). *What is dementia?* https://www.alzheimers.org.uk/sites/default/files/2018-10/400%20What%20is%20dementia.pdf

World Health Organization. (2019). *Providing everyday care* (iSupport For Dementia, pp. 107–164). World Health Organization. https://www.jstor.org/stable/resrep27895.9

## REFERENCES

Barresi, M., Ciurleo, R., Giacoppo, S., Cuzzola, V. F., Celi, D., Bramanti, P., & Marino, S. (2012). Evaluation of olfactory dysfunction in neurodegenerative diseases. *Journal of the Neurological Sciences, 323*(1–2), 16–24.

Baumgart, M., Snyder, H. M., Carrillo, M. C., Fazio, S., Kim, H., & Johns, H. (2015). Summary of the evidence on modifiable risk factors for cognitive decline and dementia: A population-based perspective. *Alzheimer's & Dementia, 11*(6), 718–726.

Livingston, G., Huntley, J., Sommerlad, A., Ames, D., Ballard, C., Banerjee, S., ... & Mukadam, N. (2020). Dementia prevention, intervention, and care: 2020 report of the Lancet Commission. *The Lancet, 396*(10248), 413–446.

Snowdon, D. A. (2003). Nun study. Healthy aging and dementia: Findings from the Nun Study. *Annals of Internal Medicine, 139*(5), 450–454. https://doi.org/10.7326/0003-4819-139-5_part_2-200309021-00014.

Song, S., Stern, Y., & Gu, Y. (2022). Modifiable lifestyle factors and cognitive reserve: A systematic review of current evidence. *Ageing Research Reviews, 74*, 101551.

Stern Y. (2002). What is cognitive reserve? Theory and research application of the reserve concept. *Journal of the International Neuropsychological Society, 8*(3), 448–460.

Ward, R., Rummery, K., Odzakovic, E., Manji, K., Kullberg, A., Keady, J., ... & Campbell, S. (2022). Beyond the shrinking world: Dementia, localisation and neighbourhood. *Ageing & Society, 42*(12), 2892–2913.

# 3

---

## PLANNING FOR THE FUTURE: WHAT ABOUT ADVANCE CARE DIRECTIVES AND CARE PLANNING?

### HOW CAN I ENSURE THAT THE WISHES OF EACH PERSON WITH DEMENTIA ARE CONSIDERED, BOTH NOW AND IN THE FUTURE WHEN COMMUNICATION MAY BECOME MORE DIFFICULT?

Planning for the future, particularly when it comes to advance care directives and care planning for a person living with dementia, is crucial to ensure that the individual's well-being and that their wishes are respected. Advance care planning is an umbrella term covering the various elements that need to be addressed to ensure a future that incorporates a personal, legal, clinical, and financial plan.

Dementia is a progressive condition that affects cognition, memory, and daily functioning, making it essential to establish plans early on while the person with dementia is still capable of participating in decision-making. Too often, families leave some of the advance care planning, for example, the creation of power of attorney, too late. If the dementia has impacted cognition enough to affect the legal capacity to make decisions, the person with dementia cannot

DOI: 10.4324/9781003457138-4

legally create a power of attorney or manage their will. If a lawyer decides that the person with dementia is incapable, it can require further costly legal steps to create a power of attorney or a substitute decision-maker. It can be done, but it costs more money to do and takes more paperwork and time. To reduce stress, the first step in future planning is to have all the legal documents signed as soon as possible after a diagnosis. It is becoming more common for people to do these legal documents as they age, but not all do, and not all do so after a diagnosis of dementia.

In this chapter, we explore the importance of advance care directives and care planning, and provide some guidance on how to effectively plan for the future (Health Service Executive HSE (HSeLanD), 2023). There are a multiplicity of factors that each individual living with dementia may be thinking about, and how to enact their wishes will vary according to the person's personality, life history, family circumstances, and the symptoms that accompany their dementia.

At the core of advance care planning is respect for human rights, particularly the domains of participation and accountability (World Health Organization, 2023). Participation for persons living with dementia means that they have the right to take part in decisions that concern them. Advance care planning allows for participation in multiple domains of personal, legal, and health-related decisions if the capacity to make decisions is compromised. It is a method for ensuring participation in the future life of the person living with dementia. Accountability in the human rights framework means that persons living with dementia can exercise their rights and freedom in all aspects of their life. Advance care planning allows for this accountability to occur – it is the formal mechanism for this accountability.

Three main domains to consider in advance care planning are the personal decisions, the legal decisions, and the healthcare decisions of the person living with dementia. Within each domain, there are multiple factors to consider, and some of these are noted below as questions that people might wish to ask to help make decisions about their future in each of these domains. Each of these domains is linked; for example, many facets of personal decisions impact healthcare decisions. Although this book focuses on dementia, everyone would benefit from considering the different facets involved in advance care plans – it is never too late to engage in advance care planning, and many people add some form of an advance care plan when making formal wills.

## WHAT IS ADVANCE CARE PLANNING?

Advance care planning or directives are legal documents that outline an individual's preferences regarding their medical treatment and care should they no longer be able to communicate their wishes. These directives, such as living wills and healthcare proxies, serve as a guide for healthcare professionals and family members, ensuring that the person with dementia receives care that aligns with their values and beliefs (Mayo Clinic, 2022; Medicare Interactive, 2024). This has been reinforced by laws governing supporting decision-making with particular reference to the United Nations Convention on the Rights of Persons with Disabilities (UNCRPD). Article 12 requires everyone to have equal recognition before the law and to achieve this, the relevant supports and safeguards must be in place (Series & Nilsson, 2018).

It is crucial to have these directives in place before cognitive decline progresses to a point where decision-making capacity is compromised (Hawkins & Charland, 2020). Capacity is used in legal contexts to describe a person's ability to make decisions for themselves, and incapacity refers to when decision-making power no longer sits with the person (Moye et al., 2013). For each adult, it is critical to have the power to make decisions for themselves, and this is consistent with the World Health Organization's (WHO) human rights framework discussed earlier. Indeed, being able to make decisions for oneself is considered a fundamental human right. Taking away a person's power to make decisions for themselves is not done lightly. Some psychiatric or medical conditions can temporarily impact capacity. Dementia can also impact capacity, but it is important to stress that a diagnosis of dementia does not automatically indicate that capacity is diminished. Formal capacity assessments are involved and in many jurisdictions, a declaration of incapacity can require more than one specially designated healthcare provider to make an independent decision of compromised capacity.

After capacity is compromised, the person with dementia cannot make legal decisions. In many jurisdictions, the legal capacity for making wills (testamentary) or financial decisions is a higher bar than the legal capacity for making healthcare decisions. Frequently, however, healthcare decisions are intertwined with financial decisions. Ideally, a substitute decision-maker or power of attorney has been legally identified, and if the person with dementia lacks capacity, this person can step in to help the person living with dementia engage with advance care planning.

It is important that people consider who to nominate as their substitute decision-maker. People rely most on this substitute decision-maker when they are at their most vulnerable. Also, being a substitute decision-maker is a very hard job. A lack of clarity in the advance care directive is one of the factors that make substitute decision-making even more stressful (King et al., 2024). An ideal substitute decision-maker is a person who is trustworthy and with whom conversations about values and end-of-life preferences can occur.

## WHAT MIGHT I WANT TO INCLUDE IN AN ADVANCE CARE DIRECTIVE?

Discussions about advance care planning should cover topics such as preferred living arrangements, medical interventions, end-of-life care, and organ donation. Table 3.1 includes details that people should consider, but it is important that each person documents their decisions and shares these with the persons they trust to honour their decisions. Advance care planning documents should be regularly reviewed and updated as the disease progresses and as circumstances change.

**Table 3.1**   Questions That People Might Ask Themselves to Help with Creating an Advance Care Plan

| | |
|---|---|
| Personal Decisions | What do you value most about your mental and physical health? Some areas to consider are how you feel about your independence, privacy, ability to communicate with others, having loved ones nearby, dignity, and being able to do your hobbies. |
| | What would make prolonging your life unacceptable to you? Some specific questions to ask yourself include being kept alive by machines with no chance of survival, being in a coma with no chance of waking up, being in pain, losing privacy, not being able to communicate with others in any way. |
| | Where do you wish to live, and what might change your mind about this choice? |
| | How do you wish to live, including at the end of life? |
| | If you were nearing death, what would make you more at peace? |
| | How do you want your pets to be looked after? |
| | What should be done with your social media information, also referred to as your digital legacy? |
| | What funeral arrangements do you want? |
| Legal Decisions | How do you wish to make your will? |
| | Who should be your power of attorney or substitute decision-maker? Should this be the same person for financial and healthcare decisions, or different people? |
| | Do you need to make provisions for dependents? |
| Healthcare Decisions | Who should assist you in making decisions for your health? |
| | How involved do you want to be in healthcare decisions near the end of life? |
| | How should you communicate your healthcare wishes? |
| | Should you communicate your wishes with your primary care provider? |

In addition to advance care directives, care planning for a person with dementia involves developing a comprehensive strategy to address their evolving needs and ensure their quality of life. The primary goal is to support the individual's well-being, safety, and engagement while minimizing distress and maintaining a sense of familiarity. A multidisciplinary approach involving healthcare professionals, caregivers, and family members is vital for effective care planning.

Care planning should encompass various aspects, including medical care, daily activities, emotional and social well-being, and safety considerations. Healthcare professionals should conduct a thorough assessment of the person's physical and cognitive abilities, as well as their behavioural and psychological symptoms. Based on this assessment, an individualized care plan can be developed, outlining the necessary support and interventions.

Medical care planning involves regular check-ups, medication management, and addressing any co-existing conditions. It is crucial to have a healthcare team that specializes in dementia care and understands the unique challenges associated with the disease.

Daily activity planning focuses on providing a structured routine, incorporating meaningful and stimulating activities that promote cognitive and physical function. Modifications to the environment, such as reducing clutter and implementing safety measures, may be necessary to ensure a dementia-inclusive space.

Emotional and social well-being should be prioritized through the provision of emotional support, social interaction, and opportunities for engagement in activities that bring joy and purpose. Carers/supporters, family members, and the wider community play a vital role in maintaining social connections and providing companionship. The entire team of medical, family, and community collaborators provides the best care model (Alzheimer Scotland, 2015).

The Alzheimer Scotland (2015) care model describes eight pillars of dementia care in communities. (See https://www.alzscot .org/delivering-integrated-dementia-care-the-8-pillars-model-of -community for the image depicting this model.) At the centre of the care model is the person living with dementia and their care partner(s). A central pillar of dementia care in this model is a dementia coordinator, who is a healthcare provider who can coordinate access to all the remaining pillars of support and who can also provide care and support for the person living with dementia and their care partner. A second pillar of support is support for carers, which refers to supports for care partners and a focus on their health and well-being. Another critical pillar includes healthcare systems that provide therapeutic interventions for the symptoms of dementia, which could include not only prescribed medications but also non-pharmacologic interventions to delay deterioration, enhance daily function, and improve quality of life. The next pillar is general healthcare systems that focus on well-being and physical health. Mental healthcare and treatment is another pillar where mental health practitioners provide appropriate services to maintain mental health and well-being. Personalized support to maintain activity and engagement is another pillar in the Alzheimer Scotland care model. Community connections is another pillar focused on maintaining and developing interpersonal support networks composed of people who are helpful and supportive, and this pillar includes peer support networks. The final pillar in this model refers to the environment and the inclusion of modifications to reduce disability, enhance accessibility, and promote independence.

It is important to assess safety considerations particularly in the home environment for potential hazards, such as slippery floors or sharp objects, and implement the necessary modifications (Health Direct Australia, 2022). This may also involve implementing strategies to prevent getting lost, which can be part of a living with dementia diagnosis.

Regular reviews and adjustments to the care plan are essential to ensure its effectiveness as the disease progresses. Communication and collaboration between healthcare professionals, caregivers, and family members are key to addressing emerging needs and making necessary adaptations.

# HOW DO I COMMUNICATE THESE PLANS TO OTHERS, FOR EXAMPLE, EXTENDED FAMILY?

When creating advance care directives for someone with dementia, it is essential to involve the person themselves, if possible, in the decision-making process. This ensures that their preferences and values are respected, promoting autonomy and dignity.

Carmel reflects on the experience of decision-making with her mother:

Once Mum received her official diagnosis, she could no longer put her affairs in order as her GP refused to allow any legal documents to be prepared. Mum actually became invisible after her diagnosis, she was talked about, and decisions were made for her by everyone but herself. This included personal care and her financial affairs; she could not have any non-essentials without authorization from the courts. Family members had become so self-absorbed that they refused to see what Mum's wishes were.

I firmly believe nobody understood the diagnosis. It was a continuous battle for services and support. As the primary carer by default, I was so distraught as I felt I was failing my mother at a time when she most needed my help.

Caring for a loved one who is living with a dementia diagnosis is difficult most times, but when you are under the spotlight from medical professionals, family, neighbours, and courts it becomes a living nightmare. This is why I decided after Mum's passing, I would continue to highlight her experience and how the system had failed her. Mum knew what she wanted, and life would have been so much less stressful if she could have documented simple requests such as her wishes for her funeral and her choice of care home for a week respite each year for me to have a break in the sun. Mum's final year was non-verbal and while we communicated very well, as only 7% of communication is verbal, life would have been so much more if her wishes had been documented.

As I didn't have Mum's wishes documented, I took it upon myself to ask the local Catholic priest to visit – he spent two hours with Mum on a Friday afternoon in mid-January, the day before her birthday. And I am happy to tell you that Mum passed away Sunday evening – totally at peace and happy to go. It was a beautiful death in her own bed in my home with her family around.

Another sad experience of that same Friday, I went to Mum's GP and asked for palliative care for her, he refused as she did not have cancer. Thankfully, this is another myth that has been addressed in Ireland and everyone is entitled to palliative care.

I believe that our laws in Ireland were totally antiquated, and we were ruled by the 'Lunacy Regulation (Ireland) Act' of 1871 (ISB, 1871). But thanks to the Assisted Decision-Making (Capacity) Act, 2015 (ISB, 2015) and new Decision Support Services, no one should experience this violation of their human rights in Ireland in the future.

Meaningful engagement of the person with dementia and their family in advance care planning will require prolonged discussion, ideally one that begins not long after diagnosis. Avoiding these discussions will create more problems in the future once the person with dementia can no longer meaningfully engage in communicating their wishes and desires. The sooner the discussion is had, the more it empowers the person living with dementia to participate in their future care planning. Families tend to find having to make substitute decisions more challenging when they feel unsure about what they are doing and when they are unclear about whether they are following the wishes of the person for whom they are making decisions (Wendrich-van Dael et al., 2020). If you are having a difficult time with this conversation, consider using helpful tools such as those found at www.advancedcareplanning .ca, www.nhsinform.scot, or www.hospicefoundation.ie. Helpful tools will orientate all family members to each task, facilitate discussion, and can be used to document decisions. Some tools also discuss the use of videos to help document decisions – not all communication of care plans needs to be communicated to family in writing! Regardless of how it is communicated, the more detail the better in the advance care plan, and using helpful advance care planning tools might help each family member remember all the details of what they need to discuss.

Another important discussion to have with family is how each of you views risk – this might be more philosophical but it is important to consider, nevertheless. Some methods used to stop wandering, for example, could substantially interfere with the quality of life of the person with dementia. Reducing all risk usually requires removal of rights and freedoms. The COVID-19 pandemic and the ban on all visitors for those in residential care to avoid exposure to the virus was a poignant example. Persons living with dementia should discuss how much they wish to balance risk with quality of life. Making decisions for a loved one that could increase their risk, for example, the risk of falling or going out walking and getting lost, is hard for families to do. It will be easier for them to do if you have all shared your beliefs on quality of life and risk, and made this important discussion part of your advance care planning. Of course, wishes may change over time and how to accommodate these is important to consider.

As Phyllis reflects:

    We must remember to update our care plans as our needs and our symptoms change. As an example, I have it written down that there are to be no feeding tubes, but when I wrote this I was only thinking of end of life. I did not consider that I may develop a swallowing disorder when I was still able to do things, be involved, and active. Now I am having to rethink this. Am I getting adequate nutrition and being able to take my medication? Would a feeding tube help to keep me enjoying my life at this point? Developing a swallowing disorder alongside my dementia while I am still fit and able has challenged me to think about what I would accept at different points in my journey with dementia.

Many people report that they would not be allowed to make their own decisions once a diagnosis was made. Unfortunately, they were at the mercy of family or whoever was seen as the official person to inherit, particularly a farm or indeed a residence. Thankfully, this is a changing situation as countries have introduced new legislation. For example, due to the recent change in the law in Ireland, there has been a shift in thinking about what the person living with dementia wants and believes is best, and adhering to what is best for the person. When nursing homes became more accessible in Ireland, many were admitted by their families and had no say in where they went. Private and public care homes are still very common, but since COVID-19, there are much tighter regulations and spot checks.

An interesting study, My Support Study to evaluate the booklet Family Carer Decision study, was a collaboration between six countries including Canada and Ireland (mySupport, n.d.; Bavelaar et al., 2022). It is now going forward under the In-Touch Horizon EU-funded project that will enhance the lives of people with dementia living in care homes through a multisensory care programme approach to improve their dignity and quality of life, while also supporting their families in decision-making (In-Touch, n.d.). Its primary objective is to mitigate social isolation by orchestrating tailored, group-based, multisensory Namaste activities for individuals with advanced dementia and their families. It aims to provide an opportunity to discuss prognosis and fundamental aspects of care.

This ongoing trial-led study will take place in 56 care homes across seven countries, focusing on palliative care, staff training, and improving well-being through tailored, multisensory activities for residents and their families. This will hopefully expand into the community to enhance those who wish to remain in their own homes until the end of life.

COVID-19 highlighted the importance of a living will, i.e. the patient's wishes documented, so there is no confusion or lack of clarity around what the person wants. This means that the family needs to adhere to their loved one's wishes.

In conclusion, when planning for the future, including advance care directives and care planning, it is crucial that the wishes of individuals with dementia are carefully considered. Advance care directives provide a mechanism to ensure that the wishes of the person living with dementia are respected, even when they are no longer able to communicate them. Care planning involves a multidisciplinary approach, aiming to address medical, emotional, social, and safety needs. By considering these aspects and involving the person with dementia in decision-making for as long as possible, we can provide person-centred care that upholds their dignity and well-being throughout the course of the disease.

## CHAPTER 3 RESOURCES

These selected resources are a good place to start to find accessible guides. It is not an exhaustive list nor does it cover all countries and different legal jurisdictions.

Alzheimer Association (US.). (n.d.). *Financial and legal planning for caregivers.* Retrieved March 31, 2024, from https://www.alz.org/help-support/caregiving/financial-legal-planning/legal-documents

Alzheimer Society of Canada. (n.d.). *Decision-making and respecting independence.* Retrieved March 31, 2024, from https://alzheimer.ca/en/help-support

/im-caring-person-living-dementia/providing-day-day-care/decision
-making-respecting

Alzheimer Society of Canada. (2022). *Decision-making and respecting individual choice* [PDF]. Retrieved March 31, 2024, from https://alzheimer.ca/sites /default/files/documents/Conversation-About-Decision-Making-en -Alzheimer-Society.pdf

Alzheimer Society (UK). (n.d.). *Dementia and the mental capacity act 2005.* Retrieved March 31, 2024, from https://www.alzheimers.org.uk/get -support/legal-financial/dementia-mental-capacity-act

Dementia UK. (2022). *Lasting power of attorney.* Retrieved March 31, 2024, from https://www.dementiauk.org/information-and-support/financial -and-legal-support/lasting-power-of-attorney/

Dementia UK. (2024). *Planning NOW for your FUTURE: Advance care planning.* Retrieved March 31, 2024, from https://www.dementiauk.org /information-and-support/financial-and-legal-support/advance-care -planning/

Dying With Dignity Canada. (2023). *Advance care planning kit* [PDF]. Retrieved March 31, 2024, from https://dyingwithdignity.ca/wp-content /uploads/2023/03/DWDC__2023ACPkit_EN.pdf

Irish Hospice Foundation. (2024). *Advance care planning.* Retrieved March 31, 2024, from https://hospicefoundation.ie/i-need-help/i-want-to-think -ahead/advance-care-planning/

NHS England, Dementia Team and End of Life Care Team. (2018). *My future wishes: Advance care planning (ACP) for people with dementia in all care settings* [PDF]. Retrieved March 31, 2024, from https://www.england.nhs.uk/wp -content/uploads/2018/04/my-future-wishes-advance-care-planning-for -people-with-dementia.pdf

Shared Care Committee. (n.d.). *The dementia companion handbook: A guide for supporting conversations with your healthcare team* [PDF]. Retrieved March 31, 2024, from https://alzheimer.ca/bc/sites/bc/files/documents/Dementia %20Companion%20Handbook_printable15.pdf

# REFERENCES

Alzheimer Scotland. (2012). *The 8 pillars model of community support.* https:// www.alzscot.org/delivering-integrated-dementia-care-the-8-pillars -model-of-community

Alzheimer Scotland. (2015). *Advanced dementia consultation response.* https:// www.rcslt.org/wp-content/uploads/media/Project/RCSLT/advanced -dementia-consultation-response-2-4.pdf

Bavelaar, L., McCann, A., Cornally, N., Hartigan, I., Kaasalainen, S., Vankova, H., Di Giulio, P., Volicer, L., Arcand, M., Van Der Steen, J. T.,

Brazil, K., & The mySupport study group. (2022). Guidance for family about comfort care in dementia: A comparison of an educational booklet adopted in six jurisdictions over a 15 year timespan. *BMC Palliative Care*, *21*(1), 76. https://doi.org/10.1186/s12904-022-00962-z

Hawkins, J., & Charland, L. C. (2020). Decision-making capacity. In E. N. Zalta (Ed.), *The stanford encyclopedia of philosophy* (Fall 2020). Metaphysics Research Lab, Stanford University. https://plato.stanford.edu/archives/fall2020/entries/decision-capacity/

Health Direct Australia. (2022). *Creating a calming, helpful home for people with dementia* [Text/html]. https://www.healthdirect.gov.au/creating-a-calming-home-for-people-with-dementia

HSeLanD. (2023). *Advance healthcare directive.* https://www.hse.ie/eng/about/who/national-office-human-rights-equality-policy/assisted-decision-making-capacity-act/advance-healthcare-directive/advance-healthcare-directive-interactive-final.pdf

In-Touch. (n.d.). *Home.* Improving Care for People with Advanced Dementia. Retrieved March 27, 2024, from https://palliativeprojects.eu/in-touch/

ISB. (1871). The Lunacy Regulation (Ireland) Act, 1871 https://www.irishstatutebook.ie/eli/1871/act/22/enacted/en/print.html#:~:text=An%20Act%20to%20amend%20the,%5B25th%20May%201871.%5D

ISB. (2015). Assisted Decision-Making Act (2015). https://www.irishstatutebook.ie/eli/2015/act/64/enacted/en/html

King, S., Fernandes, B., Jayme, T. S., Boryski, G., Gaetano, D., Premji, Z., ... & Holroyd-Leduc, J. (2024). A scoping review of decision-making tools to support substitute decision-makers for adults with impaired capacity. *Journal of the American Geriatrics Society.* https://doi.org/10.1177/1471301218802127

Mayo Clinic. (2022). *Your guide to living wills and other advance directives.* Mayo Clinic. https://www.mayoclinic.org/healthy-lifestyle/consumer-health/in-depth/living-wills/art-20046303

Medicare Interactive. (2024). *Health care proxies.* Medicare Interactive. https://www.medicareinteractive.org/get-answers/planning-for-medicare-and-securing-quality-care/preparing-for-future-health-care-needs/health-care-proxies

Moye, J., Marson, D. C., & Edelstein, B. (2013). Assessment of capacity in an aging society. *American Psychologist, 68*(3), 158.

mySupport. (n.d.). *Supporting care home staff to engage in decision-making with family carers: Scaling up an educational intervention.* Retrieved March 27, 2024, from https://mysupportstudy.eu/

Series, L., & Nilsson, A. (2018). Article 12 crpd: Equal recognition before the law. In I. Bantekas, M. A. Stein, & D. Anastasiou (Eds.), *The UN convention on the rights of persons with disabilities: A commentary.* Oxford University Press. http://www.ncbi.nlm.nih.gov/books/NBK539188/

Wendrich-van Dael, A., Bunn, F., Lynch, J., Pivodic, L., Van den Block, L., & Goodman, C. (2020). Advance care planning for people living with dementia: An umbrella review of effectiveness and experiences. *International Journal of Nursing Studies*, *107*, 103576.

World Health Organization. (2023, December 1). *Human rights*. WHO. https://www.who.int/news-room/fact-sheets/detail/human-rights-and -health#:~:text=Health%20and%20human%20rights&text=Freedoms%2 0include%20the%20right%20to,relevant%20for%20persons%20with%20 disabilities)

# Part 2

# 4

---

# HOW CAN WE PROMOTE AND MAINTAIN SOCIAL HEALTH AND WELL-BEING WHEN LIVING WITH DEMENTIA?

Psychosocial approaches offer a way to enhance living with dementia (in a context where there is no cure and only limited advances from 'big pharma' in treatments for dementia and even fewer advances in finding the ever-elusive 'cure' for dementia). If we focus on improving social or psychological well-being and health for those diagnosed and living with dementia, the focus becomes one that promotes creativity and what *can* be done, rather than a focus on a lack of abilities. Thinking about social health and well-being can encourage staff and the family to maintain relationships with the person with the diagnosis. If we consider how to promote social health and well-being, it encourages us to focus on how we can work to achieve the participation, inclusion, and involvement of people living with dementia (PLWD).

There has been a lack of funding for psychosocial work to support living well with dementia in comparison to the resources given to pharmaceutical interventions. It is a challenge in terms of how we can address this to ensure that those living with dementia are given access to opportunities to maintain their social health and well-being.

DOI: 10.4324/9781003457138-6

Psychosocial interventions or initiatives on dementia are interventions involving interaction between people to improve psychological and/or social functioning. This can include initiatives designed to improve well-being and cognition; initiatives to promote or maintain relationships with family members, other people living with dementia, and within the community; and initiatives focusing on a range of different activities that can help maintain, relearn, or learn new daily living skills – these can be as varied as cooking to learning how to use technology to maintain contact with others. A challenge that faces those working in the area is how to ensure that good local projects can help to build the overall evidence base for those working to promote social health and well-being to be able to access, draw on, and adapt to the particular group or individual they might be trying to support.

A real challenge is how to maximize the benefits for all people living with dementia, no matter what country or setting they might be living in. As has been noted: 'if psychosocial interventions have positive and cost-effective outcomes on cognition and quality of life and on rates of institutionalization, there is potential for dissemination and wider implementation' (Moniz-Cook et al., 2011, p. 286).

InterDem (https://interdem.org/) is a Pan-European network of researchers working in the social health and well-being arena of dementia studies. The second InterDem manifesto was published in 2021 (Vernooij-Dassen et al., 2021; 2019 manifesto) and moved from the original manifesto of 2011, where psychosocial was the primary focus, towards bridging biomedical and psychosocial approaches.

The six new calls within the 2019 manifesto are

1. Work on approaches and concepts at the interface of biomedical and psychosocial approaches.
2. Recognition of social health as a specific area for development.
3. Development of models of co-production in dementia research.
4. Harnessing the power of new technology for the benefit of people with dementia.

5. Interventions need to be individualized.
6. Greater attention to the implementation of research findings.

The work of the InterDem network provides a cohesive evidence base and logic to focusing on the social health and well-being of those living with dementia while recognizing the biomedical aspects of dementia (Droes et al., 2017; Vernooij-Dassen et al., 2018). What does this mean in practice for individuals seeking to support those living with dementia to maintain their social health and well-being? And what does this mean in practice for those living with a diagnosis of dementia?

The first commonly heard question is

## WHAT CAN I DO TO HELP THE PERSON LIVING WITH DEMENTIA STAY ENGAGED?

Remaining engaged with everyday activities, as well as activities focusing on hobbies and other interests, and also spending time with family and friends and remaining active in the wider community, is really important. People living with dementia report feeling better when they have the opportunity to do things they enjoy and be with other people. Retaining day-to-day skills and abilities in the home, whether that be cooking, doing the laundry, gardening, or household chores, is one way to stay engaged in the daily life of the person's own home. The activities people may engage in will differ based on their preferences, hobbies, and prior connections. What might be important for one person, for example, going to a place of worship each week or getting out for a walk every day, might be things that the person has always done. Trying to maintain routines, whether that is a weekly activity or a daily outing, is important; this allows for connections to be made to groups, the neighbourhood, and community, and provides an opportunity to get out of the house. Having the opportunity to talk to other people and to be included in family get-togethers or social meetups with friends is also important to help the person remain connected with others. There are many groups that might be suitable for the person living with dementia. Peer support groups or group activities designed for people living with dementia to get together and meet others in a similar position and experiencing similar issues can be a way to remain engaged, as people share their tips to remain active in their homes, communities, and social circle.

Another question that all those providing support to people living with dementia often ask, as well as the person living with dementia themselves, is

## WHAT CAN HELP SOMEONE TO LIVE WELL WITH DEMENTIA – FOR EXAMPLE HOW TO MINIMIZE RISK FACTORS AND MAXIMIZE PROTECTIVE FACTORS?

The lifestyle factors that help to reduce dementia risk also help to mitigate the risk of accelerated cognitive decline with non-pharmacological lifestyle interventions (Livingston et al., 2020). Perhaps one of the most important things one can do after being diagnosed with dementia is manage cardiovascular risk factors. In a clinical context, an important part of managing cardiovascular risk factors includes proper medication management to avoid missing doses of important medications or inappropriately taking multiple doses. Supervision of medication management by care partners or formal in-home care can be helped with bubble-packing medications for ease of management by persons living with dementia and for supervision by informal or formal care partners.

Engaging in physical activity and exercise is an important lifestyle activity to reduce the risk of further decline and to manage cardiovascular risk factors. Engaging in physical activity and exercise has been shown to maintain the volume of the hippocampal formation – the part of the brain involved in memory – for persons diagnosed with Alzheimer's disease (Intlekofer & Cotman, 2013). In general, engaging in physical activity and exercise has been shown across many studies with many different samples of people with dementia to be beneficial for those who have been diagnosed with dementia (Livingston et al., 2020). Engaging in social activity is also beneficial, likely because it helps to minimize depression and because it is cognitively stimulating. Minimizing symptoms of depression and engaging in cognitively stimulating activities are also important for people with dementia (Livingston et al., 2020).

To maintain quality of life, engaging in some of the lifestyle factors noted above, such as physical activity and exercise, or cognitively stimulating activities, will require balancing risk and safety. Anecdotes from a context suggest that a solution that works well is joint engagement in physical activity and exercise by persons living with dementia with their care partners. Everyone benefits from physical activity and exercise, and each benefits from the socialization that can occur when exercising together. Some people living with dementia report enjoying engaging in group exercise sessions when these have been designed to be inclusive spaces for people living with dementia, such as the Minds in Motion® (https://www.cabhi.com/completed-project-summaries/minds-in-motion-a-fitness-and-social-activity/) programmes that are available in some areas.

Getting outside is something that is important to many people. The risk of getting lost is one that family members and the person living with dementia report fearing. Simple techniques such as creating a 'safe zone' where the person is familiar and can find their own way home can work. Ensuring the person has their mobile phone and can continue to use it to call if they need assistance can also help if there are times when getting lost or forgetting how to get back home starts to become a problem. However, technologies like simple off-the-shelf tracking devices might enable the person living with dementia to go out unaccompanied to local places, like the corner shop, a well-known walk, or to get the bus into town. The technology allows them to be tracked if they get lost or to press a button to ask for assistance and to be found. An even simpler initiative that many areas have is to wear a bracelet or carry a card with an emergency number for others to call if they find the person and they are unable to call themselves. It is important to consider how risks can be taken if the person's quality of life will be enhanced by continuing to do something and what protective measures can be put in place to mitigate the risk. People living with dementia may forget to do things like turn off a tap when preparing food or washing up, or forget to turn off the hob after cooking. Many devices are available to turn off appliances automatically after a certain amount of time has passed. Simple technologies can assist in minimizing the risks that family members or the person living with dementia might encounter, e.g. risk of water damage or burning themselves (or the food left on the hob). This enables everyone, the person with the diagnosis and their family members, to feel more at ease when it comes to potentially risky situations.

---

Phyllis found the following helpful to mitigate the risks associated with her dementia progressing:

One of the first things we did in our household after I was diagnosed was to install an alarm system within the house, which included smoke, fire, and water alarms. It also included an announcer that would alert and announce door alarms. The reasoning behind this was that I was a person who didn't sleep well and was frequently up at night; what might happen if I got confused and went out? At least the alarm going off would alert my husband. Another thing we did was to obtain a medical alert bracelet that states I have Alzheimer's and has my husband's name and contact information on it. I love to shop but was afraid of overspending, so a quick trip to the bank to put a spending limit on my credit and bank card still allows me that pleasure without worry.

---

Many care partners share stories with their clinicians about sleeping lightly or with one eye open to help monitor their loved one during the nighttime, and the use of technology such as that described by Phyllis can be helpful. Anecdotes from clinical practice of the resourceful use of technology include installing door alarms to alert in-home care partners about the opening of all exterior doors or just bedroom doors. There are anecdotal stories of care partners using in-home technologies such as video conferencing to observe their loved one with dementia from another room to help mitigate some wandering behaviours.

Travelling to different countries on holidays, such as a family beach holiday, can include additional risks, but engaging in a family holiday can be worth the risks because of the benefits for quality of life. Some successful methods for taking holidays have been described anecdotally in clinical practice and include personalized hats or T-shirts with instructions on how to help find care partners in the event that the person living with dementia is separated from their family. One care partner had matching shirts created with instructions for strangers to use to help make a beach holiday possible. People living with dementia may forget to do things, for example, turn off a tap when preparing food or washing up, or forget to turn off the stove after cooking. Many devices are available to turn off appliances automatically after a certain amount of time has passed. Simple technologies can assist in minimizing the risks that family members or the person living with dementia might encounter, e.g. the risk of water damage or burning themselves (or the food left on the stove). Anecdotes from a clinical context include numerous attempts at problem-solving to minimize risks. If the person living with dementia is cooking only because they need food versus for enjoyment and are having problems preparing meals that are nutritious, some families have been able to use formal services to bring in meals and disconnect the stove in the home of the person living with dementia. In areas with no formal services, some families have used a local restaurant to help ensure the person living with dementia has proper nutrition without the need to cook at home.

A frequently asked question is

## WHAT KINDS OF ACTIVITIES PROMOTE PSYCHOLOGICAL WELL-BEING?

The answer to this question varies from person to person. What might create joy in one person and promote their well-being may not be at all enjoyable for another. This is when knowledge of the person and their preferences are critical to choosing the types of activities that may promote well-being. Different people will retain different abilities, such as mobility and the ability to walk or they may still drive and get out and about on their own. Also, each individual may change their mind about things they enjoy, and certain activities that they may not have been interested in previously become treasured pastimes. The key is to be open to trying new activities, new experiences, and meeting new people. Sometimes, it isn't the activity that appears to give the most enjoyment and promote well-being but being in the company of others that promotes well-being through being part of a group or a friendship circle that promotes psychological well-being. For others, having time alone, walking in nature, meditating, reminiscing, and looking at previous achievements can promote their well-being.

Years of research have shown how non-drug-based interventions help people living with dementia, and we sometimes refer to these as psychosocial interventions because they act on the psychology of the person living with dementia and/or their socialization. A recent review by McDermott et al. (2019) of all the research data has concluded that interventions that include multiple components are the most helpful for people living with dementia. The reason this article is so important is that it is a review of reviews – the highest-quality scientific data are those that are repeated across studies and samples. Reviews of scientific studies allow us to see what findings are repeated across many different studies. A review of reviews is at an even higher level and tells us what the science says about the state of the art. The studies involved in the review of reviews by McDermott et al. (2019) considered many aspects of the lives of persons living with dementia and considered whether the interventions made any difference.

Many different types of interventions were included in the research studies reviewed by McDermott et al. (2019). One group of studies explored the impact of exercise and physical activity, including a range of activities such as aerobic exercises, strength training, seated exercise, and walking, typically for a minimum of 30 minutes once or twice weekly over the course of several weeks or months. Another group of interventions studied were cognitive interventions. The cognitive interventions included activities such as memory training, conversation, cognitive rehabilitation, and computer-based interventions. In addition to studying many different types of interventions, the reviewed research studies looked at a variety of outcomes. In other words, what impact did the interventions have on the person living with dementia? Physical outcomes were measured by studies reviewing exercise interventions, and positive effects were described in walking speed, balance, and reduced risk of falls. Cognitive outcomes were mixed. Cognitive stimulation–based interventions demonstrated consistent improvement in cognitive functioning, while cognitive training and cognitive rehabilitation showed little or no improvement. Mood outcomes were also mixed: computer-based cognitive interventions helped improve anxiety and depression; physical interventions had no impact on mood; and psychological or social interventions were inconclusive regarding their impact on mood. Research studies that used the outcomes of activities of daily living (ADL) found that physical interventions improved ADL outcomes, particularly those with a longer duration of exercise. Cognitive interventions, on the other hand, showed no improvement for ADLs. Finally, many of the intervention studies measured quality of life outcomes. Exercise was not found to be beneficial for quality of life, whereas cognitive stimulation did improve quality of life, and individually tailored activity interventions yielded the most significant improvement in quality of life. Because of the finding from the review of reviews that some interventions impacted some but not all outcomes, McDermott et al. (2019) recommended that interventions be comprised of multiple interventions (multicomponent interventions) to impact as many outcomes as possible for persons living with dementia.

Recommendations approved by the Fifth Canadian Consensus Conference on the Diagnosis and Treatment of Dementia (CCCDTD5) (Ismail et al., 2020) from their review of different activities that help support the well-being of people living with dementia are

- Exercise for persons living with dementia (93%).
- Group cognitive stimulation therapy for PLWDs (96%).
- Psychosocial and psychoeducational interventions for caregivers of PLWDs (96%).
- Development of dementia-friendly organizations/communities for PLWDs (91%).
- Use of case management for PLWDs (93%).

For the first time, the CCCDTD5 provides a set of ranked evidence-based recommendations on psychosocial and non-pharmacological interventions for people living with dementia and their care partners. These recommendations are applicable beyond Canada and aim to inform evidence-based policies and practices around activities that are supportive of living well with dementia and can promote connection for people living with dementia and their care partners.

We now turn to a further key factor, social connection, in promoting psychological well-being and social health.

## HOW DO WE MAINTAIN SOCIAL CONNECTIONS?

Different people have different ways of connecting with others. Some people live with a partner, have children nearby, and a wide extended family. Others may live alone but have family at a distance. Others may not have many, or any, family members with whom they connect. Family can be a really excellent source of support to the person living with dementia (and their care partners), and if these connections can be nurtured and maintained, and the person living with dementia continues to be included in the usual family activities, that can be one obvious way to maintain connections.

---

As Carmel notes, the importance of the family was key to supporting her mother:

I had very little support from immediate family. This was for various reasons, including mental health, inheritance issues, and no one willing to commit to help share the care responsibility.

While many families work hard to support their loved ones, there are some who, unfortunately, do not.

Many are unable to put their differences aside to care for their loved ones, usually a parent. Of course, in many countries, including Ireland, many have emigrated and give their opinions from afar on how best to provide care.

Family dynamics are always an issue – in Ireland, we also have many individuals who have no immediate family nearby and are maybe dependent on nieces or nephews to organize their care package from afar.

It is important in rural communities to engage with various groups that provide volunteers to visit or do shopping; some arrange transportation to medical appointments. In my own experience, I relied on friends to support me with my Mum's care – my siblings were in denial of Mum's diagnosis due to a lack of understanding or conveniently overlooking the difficulties Mum and I faced on a day-to-day basis. We had a designated number of hours for a home care package which only covered personal care. While this was much appreciated, it

> also caused some stress within our routine. As you can imagine, Mum may not have wanted to get up at the time the carer came or be put under a shower and washed. There was no grey area – it also depended on the healthcare person and their relationship with Mum. Not all connected; a person with a dementia diagnosis can decide if they like someone or not. We must realize that we are letting this stranger into our home; if we feel uncomfortable, we should have the right to stop this and not feel judged.

If the person does not have family, then friends, neighbours, and community encounters will be important to maintaining social connections. For both those with and without family support, ensuring that the people around know about the dementia diagnosis and the challenges that the person experiences can be very helpful, as it enables others to understand and support the person living with dementia. This can be achieved through talking to people, sharing weblinks and other written information, and through initiatives such as Dementia Friendly or Inclusive Communities, all of which help to raise awareness about dementia and some of the issues that an individual living with dementia may experience.

For individuals who, for whatever reason, have a very limited social network, finding new groups to join and attending neighbourhood and other local events may help promote a sense of social connection. Participating in community life, going to the library, attending community meetings, and going to a local coffee shop or café all help retain connections with others.

Dementia-specific services, groups, and support are also available. Joining groups where one can meet with peers and be supported by others who are knowledgeable about dementia can be really useful for forming social connections. The resource list provided at the end of this book suggests starting points to consider for finding out more about what might be available in your country or area.

It is unfortunate that many people living with dementia, their care partners, and supporters often report isolation and a lack of support from others once the person has been diagnosed or as their dementia progresses. This gives rise to a really important final question for this chapter:

## HOW DO WE EXTEND OUR SOCIAL NETWORK?

Dementia-specific services, groups, and supports are an obvious thing to try. However, not all groups will be enjoyed by everyone. Not being put off by one group or experience, and trying another until one that is enjoyable is found, takes energy and perseverance. However, it can really pay off in terms of growing new friendships, interests, and networks. Joining one group can lead to hearing about other opportunities and activities that otherwise might not have been known, which is something regularly reported by both care partners and people living with dementia.

As we age, our friendship groups may shrink as people die, move away, or become unable to participate in activities once done together. Similarly, siblings or partners may develop health issues or die, and children may move away and be at a distance. Online connections are valuable for maintaining relationships with those who are far away, or, as we found during the COVID-19 pandemic, when it is not possible to meet in person for other reasons. Taking a class and learning to use FaceTime, Zoom, WhatsApp, or other popular apps and platforms might be worth investing the time and effort. This not only enables connections to be maintained with those already known, but also allows us to create connections with new people through online chat groups. Finding strategies to grow friendships is important and has been given attention by researchers as an area in and of itself (Ward et al., 2011; Genoe et al., 2022) and has also been discussed as a benefit arising from participating in different social groups (e.g. Smith et al., 2021).

Joining a local club – might lawn bowls be your thing? Or golf? Or bridge? Or a sewing bee? Or a community garden? Or a music group? Thinking about what you might enjoy and what support you might need to participate might be challenging initially, but pays rich rewards as new friendships are forged and new skills are learnt, or existing skills are put to good use.

Phyllis found the following helpful:

Soon after receiving my diagnosis, I joined the Alzheimer Society and took some education classes there with other people who were also newly diagnosed. After those classes were done, I joined a support group at the Alzheimer Society and really enjoyed it, so I continued to look around to see what else was out there for people with Alzheimer's or early-onset dementia. I joined other groups, like the Ontario Advisory Group, which is a group of people who work together to make changes for people living with dementia in Ontario. I also joined the Dementia Alliance International. While I was with them, I helped run support groups for people living with dementia. I found this really helpful because you were with people like yourself, so you felt comfortable and you learnt from each other. It is a way to find out if somebody's having trouble with one thing, and you may be having trouble with it too but not know how to handle it. You could listen to how they dealt with it and implement it into your life and vice versa – it was really, really helpful. Some of the things I learnt were simple. For example, I was having trouble doing laundry because when I went down to the basement to put it in, I would come upstairs and get busy with something else and forget that I was doing laundry! You know, I'd go down a week later to do more laundry and, lo and behold, there's a mess in my washer from last week's laundry! So I learnt to take yellow sticky notes, and every time I put a load in the washer, I'd write 'check washer' and when I came upstairs, I'd put it on my microwave and set the timer so that when the timer went off and I went to the microwave, sure there was nothing in there, but there was a note that said to 'go check washer'. Some of the other things I learnt were very simple. Many people don't realize that I had trouble with my language skills and writing things down on paper. I knew what I wanted to say, but they taught me how to use the voice recognition software or the microphone part of my iPad so I could speak what I needed to put into words on paper. This all helped build up my confidence to the point where I became involved in research, and I absolutely love it! The other thing I'd like to point out is that you can still travel. Although it may have to be done a little differently, you can do it with support. For me, there's nothing better than going away on a trip. A lot of times it's just my husband and I, but more recently my husband, myself, my brother and his girlfriend, and my sister and her boyfriend all went away and spent a week on the beach together. This truly brought us closer together. They were able to see that I'm still the same person, and I still enjoy the same things. Although I'm still able to do these things, while travelling there's certain things I have to put in place. When checking in for a flight, I let them know that I have Alzheimer's and that it would be helpful if I could board before anybody else so that I can get settled in before the commotion starts. And generally, they allow that and it just makes travelling so much easier for me.

By considering the above questions, you will begin to travel the path to thinking about how to improve the social health and well-being of yourself if you have dementia, or the person/people for whom you provide support and care. It can be frustrating if groups are not available that meet the interests of a person, or if social connections fade away with the progression of dementia. But there are so many different things to try that it should be possible to help maintain the social health and well-being of everyone living with dementia, if we persist and don't give up.

Promoting a dementia-inclusive society has been recognized internationally as important through initiatives designed to support dementia-friendly communities (Alzheimer Disease International, 2017). Also important is raising public awareness of dementia (WHO, 2012) through engaging with the public and explaining that with a little support, people with a diagnosis can stay engaged and active, be it in sports or other various activities, and that their opinions and lifelong learning are so valuable. Intergenerational projects are very powerful and need to be developed and supported within communities. Such approaches may help to address changes in the structure of the modern family in many countries where people may no longer benefit from multigenerational living or intergenerational connections from extended families of the past. This means that much history, folklore, traditions, and customs are being lost that could potentially support the health and well-being of people living with dementia.

# CHAPTER 4 RESOURCES

These selected resources are a good place to start to find accessible guides. It is not an exhaustive list nor does it cover all countries and different legal jurisdictions.

Administration for Community Living. (n.d.). *Living well with dementia in the community*. ElderCare.gov. Retrieved March 31, 2024, from https://eldercare.acl.gov/public/resources/brochures/docs/Living%20Well%20with%20Dementia%20in%20the%20Community.pdf

Alzheimer's New Zealand. (2016). *Living well with dementia: A guide for people diagnosed with dementia*. Retrieved March 31, 2024, from https://cdn.alzheimers.org.nz/wp-content/uploads/2021/04/Booklet-2-Living-well-with-dementia-1.pdf

Alzheimer Scotland. (n.d.). *Living well with dementia.* Retrieved March 31, 2024, from https://www.alzscot.org/sites/default/files/documents/0003/2782/Living_well_with_Dementia_Text_6021.pdf

Alzheimer's Society. (2022). *The activities handbook.* Retrieved March 31, 2024, from https://www.alzheimers.org.uk/sites/default/files/2020-11/AS_77AC_The-Activities-Handbook.pdf

Alzheimer Society of Canada. (2008). *Heads up for healthier living. Alzheimer society.* Retrieved March 31, 2024, from https://alzheimer.ca/sites/default/files/documents/Heads-Up-for-Healthier-Living-Alzheimer-Society.pdf

Alzheimer Society of Canada. (n.d.). *I'm living with dementia. Living well with dementia.* Retrieved March 31, 2024, from https://alzheimer.ca/en/help-support/im-living-dementia/living-well-dementia

Alzheimer Society of Canada. (2015). *Meaningful engagement of people with dementia.* Retrieved March 31, 2024, from https://alzheimer.ca/sites/default/files/documents/meaningful-engagement-of-people-with-dementia.pdf

NHS Education for Scotland. (2020). *Promoting psychological wellbeing for people with dementia and their carers: An enhanced practice resource.* Retrieved March 31, 2024, from https://www.nes.scot.nhs.uk/media/zw0o3utc/promoting-psychological-wellbeing-for-people-with-dementia.pdf

Ontario CLRI. (2020). *A guide to virtual creative engagement for older adults.* Retrieved March 31, 2024, from https://clri-ltc.ca/files/2021/01/A-Guide-to-Virtual-Creative-Engagement-for-Older-Adults_Feb1.pdf

# REFERENCES

Alzheimer Disease International. (2017). *Dementia friendly communities: Global developments* (2nd ed.). https://www.alzint.org/u/dfc-developments.pdf

Dröes, R. M., Chattat, R., Diaz, A., Gove, D., Graff, M., Murphy, K., Verbeek, H., Vernooij-Dassen, M., Clare, L., Johannessen, A., Roes, M., Verhey, F., Charras, K., van Audenhove, C., Casey, D., Evans, S., Fabbo, A., Franco, M., Gerritsen, D.,... Zuidema, S. (2017). Social health and dementia: A European consensus on the operationalization of the concept and directions for research and practice. *Aging and Mental Health, 21*(1), 4–17. https://doi.org/10.1080/13607863.2016.1254596

Genoe, M. R., Fortune, D., & Whyte, C. (2022) Strategies for Maintaining Friendship in Dementia. *Canadian Journal on Aging, 41*(3), 431–442. https://doi.org/10.1017/S0714980821000301

InterDem. (n.d.). Interdem website. https://interdem.org/

Intlekofer, K. A., & Cotman, C. W. (2013). Exercise counteracts declining hippocampal function in aging and Alzheimer's disease. *Neurobiology of Disease, 57,* 47–55.

Ismail, Z., Black, S. E., Camicioli, R., Chertkow, H., Herrmann, N., Laforce Jr. R., Montero-Odasso, M., Rockwood, K., Rosa-Neto, P., Seitz, D., Sivananthan, S., Smith, E. E., Soucy, J. P., Vedel, I., & Gauthier, S. (2020). Recommendations of the 5th Canadian Consensus Conference on the diagnosis and treatment of dementia. *Alzheimer's and Dementia: The Journal of the Alzheimer's Association.* https://doi.org/10.1002/alz.12105

Livingston, G., Huntley, J., Sommerlad, A., Ames, D., Ballard, C., Banerjee, S., Brayne, C., Burns, A., Cohen-Mansfield, J., Cooper, C., Costafreda, S. G., Dias, A., Fox, N., Gitlin, L. N., Howard, R., Kales, H. C., Kivimäki, M., Larson, E. B., Ogunniyi, A., Orgeta, V., Ritchie, K., Rockwood, K., Sampson, E. L., Samus, Q., Schneider, L. S., Selbæk, G., Teri, L., & Mukadam, N. (2020, Aug 8). Dementia prevention, intervention, and care: 2020 report of the Lancet Commission. *Lancet. 396*(10248), 413–446.

McDermott, O., Charlesworth, G., Hogervorst, E., Stoner, C., Moniz-Cook, E., Spector, A., ... & Orrell, M. (2019). Psychosocial interventions for people with dementia: A synthesis of systematic reviews. *Aging & Mental Health, 23*(4), 393–403.

Moniz-Cook, E., Vernooij-Dassen, M., Woods, B., Orrell, M., & Interdem Network. (2011). Psychosocial interventions in dementia care research: The INTERDEM manifesto. *Aging & Mental Health, 15*(3), 283–290. https://doi.org/10.1080/13607863.2010.543665

Smith, S., Innes, A., & Bushell, S. (2021). Music making in the community with people living with dementia and care partners – 'I'm leaving feeling on top of the world'. *Health and Social Care in the Community, 30*(1), 114–123.

Vernooij-Dassen, M., Moniz-Cook, E., & Jeon, Y. -H. (2018). Social health in dementia care: Harnessing an applied research agenda. *International Psychogeriatrics, 30*, 775–778.

Vernooij-Dassen, M., Moniz-Cook, E., Verhey, F., Chattat, R., Woods, B., Meiland, F., Franco, M., Holmerova, I., Orrell, M., & de Vugt, M. (2021). Bridging the divide between biomedical and psychosocial approaches in dementia research: The 2019 INTERDEM manifesto. *Aging & Mental Health, 25*(2), 206–212, https://doi.org/10.1080/13607863.2019.1693968

Ward, R., Howarth, M., Wilkinson, H., Campbell, S., & Keady, J. (2011). Supporting the friendships of people with dementia. *Dementia, 11*(3), 287–303. https://doi.org/10.1177/147130121421064

World Health Organization. (2012). *Dementia: A public health priority.* https://iris.who.int/bitstream/handle/10665/75263/9789241564458_eng.pdf?sequence=1

# 5

---

# WHAT CARE AND SUPPORT IN THE COMMUNITY MIGHT BE ACCESSED?

The 'event' of diagnosis is a critical point, not only for the person and their family but it is also key to providing information about the support and services available that they might require in the future. Finding out about the support available in a particular local area can be challenging. This may be due to different organizations offering different support, and waiting lists – even before the initial assessment by that service as to whether they feel that they can be of benefit to the person living with dementia. This means that when a person asks for help, it is not immediately available. We need to acknowledge that different people will be able to access different care and support depending on what is available where they live and the private resources they may have to draw on when formal services are not available; therefore, there is no universal support available across countries. However, the first step to accessing support is often an assessment and it is to this issue we first turn.

## HOW CAN DIFFERENT SUPPORTS BE ACCESSED?

To access support and services, often an assessment is first required. Such assessments often look at the age, medical history, and the

DOI: 10.4324/9781003457138-7

dementia diagnosis, but this, of course, only provides part of the picture about the situation of the person living with dementia (and their family members). Any support and care services need to be thought about in relation to the person's strengths and abilities, and who may be currently able to provide support within the immediate circle of family and friends. Sometimes, it is assumed that if the person with the diagnosis has a family member at home with them, that family member will be able to step in and help. However, that family member may have their own challenges and will not always be able to provide the support required. Different people will experience their condition differently and adopt different resources and strategies to try and compensate for any issues they may be experiencing. Emotions may be running high for both the person diagnosed with dementia and their care partner and family members. Initiatives to assist the person living with dementia and their family members to plan together have been tried; however, key elements of care pathways have been identified as problematic due to inconsistent understandings and use within, and across, countries (Orsulic-Jeras et al., 2019; Samsi & Manthorpe, 2014).

The assessment process that may come before being able to access services can be a difficult one. People living with dementia tell us that practitioners can make assumptions or not have enough time or knowledge to really ensure that the views and opinions of the person living with dementia are taken into account. Addressing the different care and support needs of those with dementia and their families often requires involving an extensive and complex network of family, friends, and neighbours, as well as health and social care services. These services may be provided by healthcare, social care, or the voluntary sector. Services may not be joined up, meaning that a person may need multiple assessments to access the different supports they require. This can be a frustrating time, as the person and/or their family may not request support until they find things too difficult and need support immediately. But the support may not be available within the timescales that the person living with dementia requires.

National dementia strategies in different countries have placed an emphasis on the need for assessment as a mechanism to support access to care and support (Vinay & Biller-Andorno, 2023). Many countries, e.g. the UK (see Alzheimer Society, 2021), have developed what are known as 'care pathways' to try and make the process of accessing support easier for all concerned, and for information on supports to be easily accessible following an initial assessment, which can then be used by all organizations to help them support each individual living with dementia. In this way, a comprehensive assessment could be shared that avoids repeating questions that the person living with dementia and their care partners are asked.

Shared assessments:

- Seek information once.
- Are led by one professional.
- Produce a single assessment of need.
- Can be used to directly access identified health and social care services (without the need for further assessment).

The benefits of shared assessment for the person living with dementia include:

- Minimizes duplication.
- Focuses on their needs, not services.
- Provides one key professional contact.
- Provides coordinated and seamless access to services and support.

For practitioners it should:

- Minimize duplication.
- Integrate systems and processes.
- Reduce bureaucracy.
- Facilitate more effective use of resources.
- Support and build on good practices.

Care pathways aim to make it clear to everyone involved what support might be available depending on the assessed needs of an individual living with dementia. In this way, there can be transparency in terms of the supports available to people living in a particular area. But the assessment also needs to avoid a 'one approach fits all' type model, as different people will have different physical and social support needs and will require flexible approaches to best meet their needs. An inconvenient truth is that if you start with an economic model, you will finish with an economic model. If you start with the care needs of the person living with dementia, then a care model should ensue.

This means that the assessment shifts from one of budget constraints to one of possibility that aligns with the needs of the individual. Such an approach would also help to address potential assessment biases that the person living with dementia may encounter when trying to access support. Practitioners may have unconscious or conscious biases that shape their approach to assessment, and the services and organizations that they suggest might help address the needs of the person living with dementia. For example, if one sees dementia from the perspective of a social model of disability or from a biomedical approach, this is likely to shape their collective social and professional response to people living with dementia, from the language they use, the assumptions they make, and the care they believe could be suitable. People living with dementia could be viewed from a biomedical perspective as irretrievably ill, progressively incapable, and fundamentally different from able-bodied, healthier, younger people, or from a disability perspective as people whose social inclusion and quality of life can be addressed at biographical, environmental, physical, and psycho-social levels. These differing assumptions may lead to very different support interventions. For example, in relation to challenging behaviour, someone who displays aggressive behaviour might experience very different approaches to their behaviour depending on the stance taken by the professional – taking a biomedical position, the person might be given sedative or anti-psychotic medication, whereas taking a psycho-social position,

**Table 5.1** Assessing and Implementing Care Needs

| Assessing | | Implementing |
|---|---|---|
| Identifying support needs | <-> | Explaining needs to providers |
| Discussing options in providers/ types of services | <-> | Upholding realistic preferences |
| Determining preferences in the way the service may be provided | <-> | Agreeing specifics of the care plan |
| Checking out possibilities with potential providers | <-> | Key information |
| Arranging viewing visits | <-> | Completing forms and introductions |

professionals might explore the underlying reasons for this behaviour and try to address these first. Table 5.1 summarizes aspects of the assessment process and how it may be implemented.

## HOW CAN WE WORK TOWARDS ENSURING THAT THE SUPPORT MEETS THE NEEDS FROM THE PERSPECTIVE OF THE PERSON LIVING WITH DEMENTIA?

How to include the views of the person living with dementia in developing appropriate care and support choices has been the source of much discussion, as summarized by Innes et al. (2021) in their review of ways to improve the inclusion of people living with dementia in decisions about their care options. Therefore, it is critical to approach assessments of support needs by focusing on what the person living with dementia and their advocates say their challenges are and their views on what might enable them to be addressed.

Phyllis reflects on the process she experienced when trying to seek support:

This has been a very difficult area for me because shortly after the diagnosis, my family doctor retired, and his son took over the practice. When this happened, I didn't have the same connection with him – it makes it hard for me because he doesn't understand me the way my old doctor did. I am very vocal and speak up for myself, and my new doctor finds that very difficult to handle, so I still have a problem getting anything done when I'm dealing with him. However, I do have a much easier time when I see the neurologist or a specialist to get things done and put in place. For example, when I started to have swallowing problems, I went to my family doctor, but he said that people with Alzheimer's don't get swallowing problems. It took me probably two years to finally get him to refer me for an assessment. It is very difficult, and I find this with anything I require when I deal with him, so I just put my head down and push for myself and I do not take no for an answer, which doesn't make our relationship any easier! But that's what I personally have to do at this point. I also stand up for myself; I do not let anybody tell me how things are to be done. They assume they know what's right for me, but they don't know, so I do speak up. As an example of this, I had to have a test done at the hospital. I had seen the specialist and signed all the paperwork, so I went to the hospital for the test. On that morning, my husband waited in the truck since he had just had his knee replaced. When I went in, the nurse was checking me in and doing her assessment, and she asked where my care partner was. I explained, and she said, 'well, if he doesn't come up, then we can't see you'. I was taken aback by that statement and, me being me, I just said 'what do you mean, you won't be able to see me or do the test?' and she said 'well that's policy', and I said, 'you better make sure you're correct, because I know you're not correct and that you're assuming because I have dementia I can't sign. I can do anything while I am fully competent to take care of myself. I do not need my care partner to do that for me, so I highly suggest that you go and speak to the doctor doing the test and get his opinion on this because if I leave here without this test today, be darn sure I'm going to be putting in a call and I will be suing you under the premise that you're infringing on my human rights to care'.

---

Carmel reflects on the importance of the inclusion of the person living with dementia in the development and implementation of a care plan:

We had no support to put this in place but had to fight daily for services and supports. I now look at models of care in other countries and compare them to my experience. I think Scotland was very innovative with their introduction of link workers, who were originally assigned for a year but now remain with the person (Alzheimer Scotland, 2023). There is now more focus on the expansion of primary care capacity, and the community nurse has more authority around decisions for their patients.

Innovative initiatives like a mobile x-ray unit will definitely make life easier (Health Service Executive, 2023). This is a great service for rural and isolated regions. It also saves our most vulnerable from the stress of having to arrange travel and attend their nearest hospital, where they may spend many hours sitting, waiting for their appointment. In Ireland, the health minister announced changes in legislation, giving pharmacists a wider scope, which again will minimize travel, stress levels, and expenses for all involved (Department of Health, 2023).

---

Polypharmacy, which is when a patient is prescribed medications for various conditions at the same time, is another issue that is slowly being acknowledged (NIH, 2021). The medications may be necessary, but the side effects and drug interactions are often harmful and result in serious follow-on effects. Highlighting the risk of taking multiple medications and drinking alcohol is also vital (Gitto et al., 2016; Rehm et al., 2019). Research demonstrates that there are ways to support the medication prescribing for people living with dementia (Hanjani et al., 2019). Simple things like regular reviews of the medications the person is taking, conducted in the primary care setting, could help to avoid some of the side effects that people living with dementia experience. However, a recent review by Sharma et al. (2023) demonstrates the paucity of such reviews being conducted for people living with dementia.

The body of evidence on supporting people living with dementia, from research and from the experiences of people living with dementia and their care partners, demonstrates that providing high-quality, appropriate support can help to reduce avoidable admissions to hospital and institutional care, and the frequent use of emergency rooms, which are high cost and also often highly stressful for the person living with dementia and their care partners (Ma et al., 2019; Williamson et al., 2021). Many people living with dementia want to continue to live at home, and ensuring that home-based supports are given higher priority is important, not only for their well-being but also to avoid crisis points that can lead to a downward cycle of increased care and support needs (Leverton & Pui Kin Kor, 2023). In a study exploring the views of stakeholders about helping people living with dementia to remain at home independently, Rapaport et al. (2020) argue that a balance between independence and the associated risk-taking that may be involved, alongside appropriate psycho-social interventions to provide high-quality support, is essential. In another review, the preferences reported of people living with dementia are to have a say in their care decisions, to avoid being a burden to others while continuing to receive the support of their family, and to ensure the care partner's well-being (Wehrmann et al., 2021). How to achieve this remains a challenge in a context where home-based supports are often limited in their availability. However, meeting this challenge is essential if we are to find a way forward to meet the wish of the majority of people living with dementia to remain in their own home for as long as possible. This means that support services need to provide support within the home and the community to avoid, or delay, the more costly and less preferred option of long-term care.

Social factors such as ageism, the dominance of rationality in Western society, stereotyping, disabling environments, and the focus on productivity and cost reduction can lead to a dynamic where the needs of the person living with dementia are not at the centre, and where a poor fit between what is available and what is required is experienced.

The first point of contact to access services is often a primary care practitioner, who can be a general practitioner (GP) or family physician, community nurse, or, if the person has managed to locate voluntary services, Alzheimer's advocacy groups and societies. However, GPs are often the first gatekeepers to support because they are most likely to be the professionals with whom family members and/or the person living with dementia will discuss their concerns. This means that the GP not only provides the start of the process to get a diagnosis but also signposts the services and supports that may be available. Many doctors are now involved in social prescribing, that is, referring to community supports such as gyms, swimming pools, and other local resources. Social prescribing has been argued to offer a benefit to the person living with dementia when they are involved in the decision-making about activities (Baker & Irving, 2016). In their systematic review of social prescribing for older adult well-being, Rapo et al. (2023) found three key factors that would enhance the success of such an approach: conducting a full assessment before prescribing, matching participants with relevant activities that met their needs and interests, and individualized support from a link worker. In essence, social prescribing was more beneficial when it had been prescribed in as much of a person-centred manner as possible. Primary care workers can also provide information about the benefits and financial supports available and may refer on to specialist services such as occupational therapy if aides are needed in the home, physical therapy if there are mobility concerns, speech and language therapy when there are issues relating to communication, and nutritionists when there are problems with retaining weight or swallowing.

Other community practitioners, such as pharmacists, may notice changes in memory or ability when a person collects prescriptions, or they may notice that there is a risk of side effects due to the combination of medications a person is taking. Staff working in other community-based organizations such as banks, post offices, and grocery stores may also notice regular customers forgetting if they have withdrawn cash or buying the same items on numerous occasions (as the person has forgotten they have already been shopping that week). The dementia-friendly community movement is encouraging the wider community to be aware of dementia and to develop appropriate strategies to address concerns they may have about regular customers, as well as ensuring their approach is inclusive of those with cognitive difficulties. In this way, there is a move towards more inclusive and capable communities (Lin & Lewis, 2015).

Dementia has implications for capacity and the ability to decide and, particularly, for the assumptions by others regarding their competency (Donnelly et al., 2019). The diagnosis of dementia does not necessarily mean that the person is unable to make the decision to remain at home; however, decisions about their future are often made by others (family members, professionals) without consideration of the wishes of the person with dementia. There is an imbalance of power here and an emphasis on risk avoidance. The person living with dementia may be concerned about their safety, and usually family members are very concerned about safety. This often means that positive risk-taking approaches can be difficult to balance with safety concerns. Risk is socially constructed; that is, what is seen as risky by one person may not be seen as risky by another. Much time and effort have been spent on developing risk tools to help professionals identify, measure, and in a way predict the hazards facing a person. Positive risk-taking acknowledges that people have to take risks to grow and, of particular relevance to dementia, to maintain their preferred lifestyle and their identity. Let's think about the risks that are involved in cooking; a safety-first approach could lead to the person being advised (or prevented) from using a hob, rather than trying to work out how the person could be supported in carrying out some cooking-related tasks. Technology can help when assessing concerns about safety. In the cooking example, there are technologies that could be implemented, for example, using simplified control knobs, introducing sensors that will automatically turn off the cooker, installing a smoke detector just in case. Positive risk-taking, where the focus is to maximize the remaining ability while minimizing risk, can be vital for the sense of worth, value, and self-identity of the person living with dementia.

Thus, another challenging issue when being assessed in relation to the support available is risk. What is seen as acceptable to one person and risky to another can be very different (Rapaport et al., 2020). The person living with dementia may be willing to take more risks than their family members are comfortable with them taking. Balancing risk with autonomy requires flexible, collaborative approaches where everyone's viewpoints are considered, but where the well-being, needs, and preferences of the person living with dementia are at the centre of the decision-making process.

Phyllis is clear in setting out her belief and expectation of being involved in her support needs:

I support us [people with the diagnosis] in being included fully in any decision-making process around our care. It is highly important to me that I have a say in my own well-being because it is my life; it is still up to me what I am willing to accept and what happens to me. There was a time when my pharmacy actually made a mistake with my medications. They were giving me a medication that the doctor had cancelled, and they knew about it. But when my monthly prescription came out the next month, they re-introduced it, and I had been taking it for quite a while before I realized that I was! So, with that, I didn't feel comfortable with them anymore, and we actually left that pharmacy. When I was looking for a new pharmacy, I interviewed my pharmacist to make sure he understood my dementia and how important it was to ensure that there are never any mistakes with my medications. We were able to find somebody that takes great care of my medications, and they call me every month to check in before they send out my prescription. The other thing that they were really good at was realizing when my swallowing was starting to become a problem. We had a discussion about how I could take my tablets, and the solution was very simple. Rather than me skipping my medications like I was starting to do, they switched it over to a liquid formula, which just makes it so much easier for me at this point! You don't want to be skipping medications. The other thing I firmly believe is that people living with dementia decline slowly, and that they should be receiving physiotherapy to keep them physically stronger and moving longer, and this doesn't happen at all. So, I make sure that I do it myself by going to exercise and doing things that keep me physically strong.

The importance of accessing support and considering what the person living with dementia wants is vital. A lack of suitable support and failure to truly consider the needs of the person living with dementia place an extra layer of tasks on family members to try and find solutions themselves, often at a time when they might be finding it difficult to support their family member and negotiate the health and social care system where they live.

Carmel did not have the best experience accessing support, and she reflects on what could have helped:

Having received the diagnosis, it would have been very helpful to have been assigned someone like a case worker or link worker, similar to the model in Scotland. It would have been such a relief to have someone to signpost the supports and services available in our area. We left the neurologist's office with no information except the diagnosis. A pack containing basic information should be available at the point of diagnosis for the person and their chosen support to refer to at a later date. Regarding risk assessment, this could change on a daily basis. I found Mum's capacity could be affected if she experienced a mini stroke – senses were primarily affected, so the temperature of liquids was difficult to monitor, and making tea or cooking at any level was a challenge. Having access to a solid fuel fire was dangerous, and I could not leave Mum in a room with a fire. In rural Ireland, driving is a big issue as losing your ability to drive really affects your independence (HSE, n.d.). In Ireland, we do a yearly driving test, and also your GP will advise if they feel your capacity has changed.

My Mum had so many falls and breaks that it was constantly difficult trying to keep her mobility strong. The local healthcare physiotherapist insisted that her declining mobility was due to the ageing process. We refused to accept this and went to a private physiotherapist, which, of course, was a 20-mile drive away and had to be self-funded. However, the difference this made to Mum's quality of life was worth it. It was more than the physiotherapy; it was Mum feeling in control, having a choice, and being more than a statistic on the healthcare list.

Thinking about an inclusive approach when assessing, planning, and implementing services and support for people living with dementia means involving the person living with dementia not only in their own support and care decisions but also generally in service provision. This includes the development, running, management, and evaluation of the service. Significantly, it is younger, physically disabled people and people with mental health problems who have led the way in this respect. It is likely that the reason why people with dementia have traditionally had less opportunity to participate in planning and delivering services stems from their historical marginalization in society, along with assumptions of incapacity in areas of decision-making. The concept of participative care in relation to dementia attempts to encourage people with dementia to be involved in decisions about their own care (Brannelly, 2004). It is collaborative; being negotiated between professionals, people with dementia, and their carers, and it attempts to make the person with dementia central to the care process. The need for assessment and access to appropriate care and support are increasingly seen as part of a human rights issue, where the person living with dementia has the right to make decisions about their own support and care (Wied et al., 2019).

## CHAPTER 5 RESOURCES

These selected resources are a good place to start to find accessible guides. It is not an exhaustive list nor does it cover all countries and different legal jurisdictions.

Alzheimer Society of Canada. (n.d.). *Programs and services.* Alzheimer Society of Ontario. Retrieved March 31, 2024, from https://alzheimer.ca/on/en/help-support/programs-services

Alzheimer's Research UK. (n.d.). *Support for people affected by dementia.* Retrieved March 31, 2024, from https://www.alzheimersresearchuk.org/wp-content/plugins/mof_bl_0.2.9/downloads/CAR-0720-0722_WEB.pdf

Dementia UK. (n.d.). *Sources of support.* Retrieved March 31, 2024, from https://www.dementiauk.org/wp-content/uploads/2023/07/dementia-uk-sources-of-support-practicalities.pdf

Ontario. (n.d.). *Making a referral: Home and community care support services.* Retrieved March 31, 2024, from https://healthcareathome.ca/making-a-referral/

United Hospital Fund. (2013). *Referring patients and family caregivers to community-based services: A provider's guide.* Retrieved March 31, 2024, from https://www.nextstepincare.org/uploads/File/Guides/Provider/Community_Based_Services.pdf

# REFERENCES

Alzheimer Society. (2021). The care needs assessment: Support for people with dementia. https://www.alzheimers.org.uk/get-support/legal-financial/dementia-care-needs-assessment

Alzheimer Scotland. (2023, February 2). *A day in the life of a post diagnostic support link worker.* https://www.alzscot.org/news/a-day-in-the-life-of-a-post-diagnostic-support-link-worker

Baker, K., & Irving, A. (2016). Co-producing approaches to the management of dementia through social prescribing. *Social Policy & Administration, 50*(3), 379–397.

Brannelly, T. (2004) *Citizenship and care for people with dementia: Summary research paper.* University of Birmingham www.socialresearch.bham.ac.uk/const.htm

Department of Health. (2023, November 6). *Minister for Health progresses enhanced role for pharmacists following first recommendation of Expert Taskforce.* https://www.gov.ie/en/press-release/a90c0-minister-for-health-progresses-enhanced-role-for-pharmacists-following-first-recommendation-of-expert-taskforce/

Donnelly, S., Begley, E., & O'Brien, M. (2019). How are people with dementia involved in care-planning and decision-making? An Irish social work perspective. *Dementia, 18*(7–8), 2985–3003. https://doi.org/10.1177/1471301218763180

Gitto, S., Golfieri, L., Caputo, F., Grandi, S., & Andreone, P. (2016). Multidisciplinary view of alcohol use disorder: From a psychiatric illness to a major liver disease. *Biomolecules, 6*(1), 11. https://doi.org/10.3390/biom6010011

Hanjani, L. S., Long, D., Peel, N. M., Peeters, G., Freeman, C. R., & Hubbard, R. E. (2019). Interventions to optimise prescribing in older people with dementia: A systematic review. *Drugs Aging, 36,* 247–267. https://doi.org/10.1007/s40266-018-0620-9

Health Service Executive. (2023, September 4). *Mobile X-ray service benefits patients and reduces ED visits.* HSE.Ie. https://www.hse.ie/eng/about/our-health-service/making-it-better/mobile-x-ray-service-benefits-patients-and-reduces-ed-visits.html

HSE. (n.d.). *MEMORY LOSS AND DRIVING.* https://www.hse.ie/eng/dementia-pathways/files/memory-loss-and-driving-a-guide-for-the-person-with-memory-problems.pdf

Innes, A., Smith, S. K., & Bushell, S. (2021). Dementia friendly care: Methods to improve stakeholder engagement and decision making. *Journal Healthcare Leadership, 13,* 183–197. https://doi.org/10.2147/JHL.S292939

Leverton, M., & Pui Kin Kor, P. (2023). Supporting people with dementia to live at home. *BMC Geriatrics, 23,* 681. https://doi.org/10.1186/s12877-023-04389-w

Ma, C., Bao, S., Dull, P., Wu, B., & Yu, F. (2019). Hospital readmission in persons with dementia: A systematic review. *International Journal of Geriatric Psychiatry, 34*(8), 1170–1184. https://doi.org/10.1002/gps.5140

NIH. (2021, August 24). *The dangers of polypharmacy and the case for deprescribing in older adults.* National Institute on Aging. https://www.nia.nih.gov/news/dangers-polypharmacy-and-case-deprescribing-older-adults

Orsulic-Jeras, S., Whitlatch, C. J., Szabo, S. M., Shelton, E. G., & Johnson, J. (2019). The SHARE program for dementia: Implementation of an early-stage dyadic care-planning intervention. *Dementia,18*(1), 360–379. https://doi.org/10.1177/1471301216673455

Rapaport, P., Burton, A., Leverton, M., Herat-Gunaratne, R., Beresford-Dent, J., Lord, K. Downs, M., Boex, S., Horsley, R., Giebel, C., & Cooper, C. (2020). "I just keep thinking that I don't want to rely on people." A qualitative study of how people living with dementia achieve and maintain independence at home: Stakeholder perspectives. *BMC Geriatrics, 20,* 5. https://doi.org/10.1186/s12877-019-1406-6

Rapo, E., Johansson, E., Jonsson, F., Hörnsten, A., Lundgren, A. S., & Nilsson, I. (2023). Critical components of social prescribing programmes with a focus on older adults - A systematic review. *Scandinavian Journal of Primary Health Care, 41*(3), 326–342. https://doi.org/10.1080/02813432.2023.2237078

Rehm, J., Hasan, O. S. M., Black, S. E., Shield, K. D., & Schwarzinger, M. (2019). Alcohol use and dementia: A systematic scoping review. *Alzheimer's Research & Therapy, 11,* 1. https://doi.org/10.1186/s13195-018-0453-0

Samsi, K., & Manthorpe, J. (2014). Care pathways for dementia: Current perspectives. *Clinical Interventions in Aging, 9,* 2055–2063. https://doi.org/10.2147/CIA.S70628

Sharma, R., Mahajan, N., Fadaleh, S. A., Patel, H., Ivo, J., Faisal, S., Chang, F., Lee, L., & Patel, T. (2023). Medication reviews and clinical outcomes in persons with dementia: A scoping review. *Pharmacy, 11*(5), 168. https://doi.org/10.3390/pharmacy11050168

Vinay, R., & Biller-Andorno, N. (2023). A critical analysis of national dementia care guidances. *Health Policy, 130*(2023), 104736. https://doi.org/10.1016/j.healthpol.2023.104736

Wied, T. S., Knebel, M., Tesky, V. A., & Haberstroh, J. (2019). The human right to make one's own choices - implications for supported decision-making in persons with dementia: A systematic review. *European psychologist*, *24*(2), 146–158.

Wehrmann, H., Michalowsky, B., Lepper, S., Mohr, W., Raedke, A., & Hoffmann, W. (2021). Priorities and preferences of people living with dementia or cognitive impairment – A systematic review. *Patient Prefer Adherence, 15,* 2793–2807. https://doi.org/10.2147/PPA.S333923

Williamson, L. E., Evans, C. J., Cripps, R. L., Leniz, J., Yorganci, E., & Sleeman, K. E. (2021). Factors associated with emergency department visits by people with dementia near the end of life: A systematic review. *Journal American Medical Directors Association, 22*(10), 2046–2055.e35. https://doi .org/10.1016/j.jamda.2021.06.012

# 6

## HOW DO I SUPPORT THE PERSON LIVING WITH DEMENTIA WITH HOSPITAL APPOINTMENTS AND ADMISSIONS?

### HOW CAN WE PREPARE FOR A PLANNED HOSPITAL APPOINTMENT TO MINIMIZE DISTRESS FOR A PERSON LIVING WITH DEMENTIA?

We all have times in our lives when we get ill. We may need to visit our family physician, a specialist, or even have a hospital admission. These visits may cause great anguish to a person living with dementia and their care partner. The challenge of creating hospital environments that are inclusive and accessible to people living with dementia has long been recognized with a focus on the experiences and challenges faced by hospital staff (Handley et al., 2017; Gwernan, 2020). Initiatives to help guide the process of hospitals working towards becoming dementia friendly, such as the Dementia Friendly Hospital Charter in the UK, help create a framework for hospitals to adhere to and thus enable them to provide a high-quality care experience for the person living with dementia (NICE, 2021). The UK charter was developed by the National Dementia Action Alliance, with hospitals encouraged to

DOI: 10.4324/9781003457138-8

sign up to a commitment to develop their care to be dementia friendly. The National Dementia Action Alliance website closed in January 2024, but provided an array of information, some of which can still be accessed via the UK Alzheimer's Society. From their review of the international literature on dementia- friendly hospitals, Manietta et al. (2022) set out the key aspects that can contribute to a hospital providing a dementia-friendly experience. Two of these factors relate to the hospital itself: valuing relatives and the knowledge and expertise of the hospital. The other four factors identified relate to patient care, described as continuity of care, person-centred care, consideration of dementia and how to provide care that is knowledgeable and takes account of the challenges that people living with dementia might face, and the physical environment of the hospital itself.

The journey through a hospital may start with a planned appointment. As each of these appointments can be very different, it is important to consider what can be done to help improve the experience. Another factor that plays a role in these appointments is the reason for seeing a particular physician or specialist. Additionally, whether a firm diagnosis of dementia has been made or whether a specialist diagnosis might be required through further tests, assessments, and appointments may also play a role.

If an individual, either the person with dementia or their care partner, has concerns and is seeing the family doctor for an initial visit either for their dementia or another condition or health concern, there are a number of things that can be prepared to try and ensure that this first appointment runs smoothly.

When making the appointment, explain why the appointment is being requested and that the person living with dementia may require more time than a usual appointment slot. By doing this, it allows the receptionist to book a time slot that accommodates the time that is needed. The other thing that may happen is that after an initial appointment to review and get an overview of the issue(s), there may be referrals for other tests and appointments with other specialist services, such as blood tests, and an appointment may then be made for further follow-up after sufficient time has been allocated for any other tests, and the results are available. When making the first and follow-up appointments, it is always good to consider the time of day of the appointment, as well as the reason for the appointment. This is important as there may be a time of day when the person for whom the appointment is made is at their best. Don't make it late in the day if they are usually tired at this time or during a time when they usually have a nap.

Carmel found that she needed to prepare in the following ways to support her mother when attending hospital appointments:

Any appointments we had were a distance away in the main urban town, so we tried to have late morning or early afternoon appointments. This did not upset Mum's morning routine and kept us relaxed and happy.

The actual trip meant packing a bag that contained a change of clothes, sanitary essentials, snacks, drinks, questions we wanted to ask, and medication. We had bought a wheelchair after the diagnosis so we would not have to stress about distances when parking.

We always arrived early to secure parking and get to the office on time. Neither Mum nor I liked to get anxious. I was always allowed to stay with Mum, even when she was having an MRI. A few medical professionals did not address Mum directly, and we both found this upsetting, but Mum would never complain or be rude.

How one prepares for a diagnostic appointment might be different from how one prepares for a general medical appointment. Regardless of the purpose of the appointment, it is a good idea to be clear about when a particular problem began (onset), how frequently this problem occurs, what the impact of this problem is on all aspects of functioning (how severe the problem is), and whether the problem is increasing or decreasing in frequency or severity (course of problems over time). Taking the example of memory problems, clinicians will ask about onset, severity, and course of problems over time. It is also good to detail past and present medical conditions and treatment for medical conditions. Clinicians will ask about all currently prescribed medications and use of non-prescribed substances, and they will ask whether medications are taken as prescribed (and find out how well families have been tracking this to be able to report on this reliably). For a diagnostic appointment, it might be helpful to speak with the diagnosing clinician alone, and if this does not seem possible, care partners can write letters detailing what symptoms they have noticed and the impact these symptoms have on functioning.

Before going to the appointment, it can be useful to take some time to gather information to take with you.

- Make a list of any concerns. For example, there are great website resources.
- Take a list of medications or pack a bag with the actual medications.
- Write out a detailed family history.
- Think about and write down any questions that have been building up about the issue.
- It is always good that someone attends the appointment with the person living with dementia so they can assist with, for example, helping find the location of the appointment, taking notes, or simply as an extra set of ears, as they may hear or understand things differently.

It is important to be prepared not to get an answer at this initial consultation. Many things need to be done before you can get an answer. It is wise to expect multiple tests and possibly multiple appointments with the family doctor or referrals to other specialists.

One of the first things a family doctor may want to do is to rule out any underlying causes. They may instruct blood tests, x-rays, or other scans, or an array of further testing. If the person (or the family member) has any questions, it is absolutely fine to ask why certain tests are being carried out to help everyone understand what is happening. It can also reduce anxiety and worry about things that may not be as important or as difficult as they might sound. If you are unsure or have questions, ask them. Don't forget to ask what, if anything, is needed to prepare for the test.

When going for tests, make sure to follow the instructions given. If, after the appointment is made and any letter is received, there are still questions about the tests, it is usually possible to call the office of the referred specialist. Medical teams prefer calls to help clarify rather than having to cancel and reschedule appointments due to a lack of preparation and understanding. It is important to avoid unnecessary delays and stress for the person living with dementia.

---

Phyllis reflects on her experience of attending an appointment with her spouse:

I would like to point out that a lot of times you are bringing your spouse with you to your appointments. However, you have to keep an eye on this because I know my husband didn't believe there was a problem with me. He hadn't seen it, and it took him quite a while before he really realized what was going on. So, he was giving his opinion that there was nothing wrong with me, while I was saying, 'well, this is going on' 'that's going on', and they weren't getting a full picture. Over the years, yes, there's times when it's been very helpful, but lately it's not. You see, my children and I are starting to think that he's developing signs and symptoms of dementia, but he's refusing to be tested. So, the way he sees things now, it's totally different, and it does make it difficult. Therefore, we need to keep an open mind. I have started to take my daughters with me to appointments rather than my husband, and I think we always have to be well aware of what's happening. This may be difficult when it's a husband and wife team who aren't involved with family or friends because somebody else isn't saying the same things we are.

Once the doctor has all the test results, they may call or request a return in-person appointment to discuss what the results suggest. It is possible that a direct referral may be made to see a specialist. Remember that every time a person living with dementia has an appointment with a new doctor or health team, the list above applies. This can help with any glitches between different people and systems sharing information.

In Ireland, dementia awareness has made great progress over the last ten years. Ireland's first and only dementia strategy was launched in December 2014 (Department of Health, 2019). It is a very slow process; probably one of the main learnings has been to put supports and services before campaigning for early diagnosis. There is still a large divide between urban and rural areas, but this is slowly being addressed. It is so important that all organizations work together and not in silos. Silos are of no benefit to the affected communities and have to be avoided. My own learning over my time being involved in advocacy is to learn from others, at home and abroad, and take your learning home to improve the quality of life for all.

An example of person-centred care and putting the person first: there is an incredible and true life-changing story from one of Ireland's old mental hospitals/homes, where a patient had been a resident for over 40 years, when a lead member of staff finally wanted to change the narrative of 'statistics' about patients and instead have her patients seen as the human beings they deserved to be.

https://youtu.be/2jEHLkrMeFg?si=GQA6oRT_eF89si-H

Here are links to websites that outline the different ways to prepare for appointments. These are from different countries but are relevant to anyone wishing to improve the life of a person living with dementia:

https://www.understandtogether.ie/

https://alzheimer.ie/living-with-dementia/i-have-dementia/first
-steps-after-diagnosis/

https://www.alzheimer-nederland.nl/dementie/diagnose-en
-behandeling

https://www.francealzheimer.org/comprendre-la-maladie/la
-maladie-dalzheimer/traitements-construire-parcours-de
-soin/

https://alzheimer.ca/sites/default/files/documents/tipsheet_pre
paringforyourdoctor_e.pdf.pdf

https://alzheimer.ca/sites/default/files/documents/getting-a-diag-
nosis-toolkit.pdf

These are suggested examples, but looking up what information is relevant to where the person is located is a good idea. There might be country-specific, hospital-specific, and procedure-specific guidelines that can be consulted to help inform how to prepare.

## WHAT SHOULD WE DO IF THERE IS AN EMERGENCY ADMISSION TO HELP HOSPITAL STAFF SUPPORT THE PERSON LIVING WITH DEMENTIA MOST EFFECTIVELY?

There may be times when someone becomes sick or hurt and may need to visit a local accident and emergency department, emergency room, or urgent care. This time can be very stressful for both the person living with dementia and their care partners. It is always best to think about how one might prepare for this well ahead of ever having to do so. This will help make the situation a little easier.

Here is a checklist of things that are useful to take if there is an emergency admission:

- Any medical cards that may be needed to enable the person to receive the required care.
- A list of emergency contacts. It may help if these are in the order of who is to be called first, second, and so on.
- A copy of the power of attorney or medical care, just in case it is needed.
- The contact details for your family doctor and any specialists.
- A list of medications.
- A detailed history relating to the different conditions.
- A list outlining why you are there now.
- Another thing you may like to take is a quick information guide about the person.
- Most importantly are any advance directives that the person may have.

This list may look long, but these are all the things you can prepare ahead of time. They will make these emergency times easier on everyone.

If an ambulance is required, make sure they have a copy of these things as it helps them care for your loved one, and they will pass it on to the hospital.

Phyllis has found the following helpful:

I keep a copy of my medical information by my front entrance, tagged for emergency medical personnel.

I actually have two envelopes, one for myself and one for my husband, and in each envelope, we keep a copy of our power of attorney. We keep a sheet of paper that has all our medical information on it, our legal names, our health card numbers, the medications we take, our emergency contacts, including their phone numbers, and a list of all our medical problems. I also keep a list in my envelope of my wants and wishes, such as my 'do not resuscitate' and 'allow a natural death', and medical treatments that I will accept and those I won't.

Carmel reflects on the difficulties she experienced as a care partner and how these led to her advocating for change:

Living in rural Ireland, if Mum had an emergency admission to hospital, I was always allowed to travel with her in the ambulance and stay with her in the emergency unit. The medical staff would note her dementia diagnosis, but unfortunately most of Mum's hospital admissions were prior to her diagnosis. Mum was having a lot of falls, and osteoporosis was diagnosed; unfortunately, the reason behind the falls was not detected ntil much later – mini stroke (Irish Osteoporosis Society, 2021; HSE, 2021).

In 2016, following my advocacy for better support, our local hospital introduced the Butterfly Scheme https://butterflyscheme.org.uk This is a very simple yet effective system, putting a butterfly symbol on the patient's chart or over their bed. The scheme was developed by a lady Barbara Hodkinson who cared for her mother. They had a bad experience during a hospital stay and she decided to campaign to improve the service. It involves training of hospital staff in all departments around how to recognise the signs of dementia, to communicate with the patient, to avoid the patient being moved from various wards, the importance of having the patient in a quiet relaxed ward near the nurse's station. The training is carried out by trained family carers and so has the benefit of the lived experience.

Patients who wish to participate are identified by a simple butterfly symbol on their chart or on their bed. It is a simple but very effective method of identifing patients with temporary confusion, delirium, temporary memory loss or dementia to be treated more effectively, this is very helpful in accident and emergency where due to delays a patients starts to experience confusion and aggitation.

Another very important issue was highlighting the importance of keeping the patient in a smaller wad and not moving them. Unfortunately, when staff move and new staff are not trained, the practice loses its efficacy.

Ireland health board service has just launched the 'Getting to Know What Matter To Me' Dementia Passport This will be an important step in making the patient experience a more personised expereince. Staff will be in a position to familarise themselves with the persons background, daily activities, likes/dislikes, family history.

Upon arrival at the hospital, it is important to share with the admission team that the person has dementia, making them aware that the person may require more time to communicate and understand. Additionally, they might feel more comfortable if they have someone from the family or a care partner with them.

This is important for two reasons, which may have to be explained to the hospital staff. The first is for comfort and to help promote the feeling of safety for the person living with dementia; and the second reason is that the staff can use this information to assist in helping the person living with dementia understand what is happening. If necessary, ask for a quiet area to help, but be aware that due to the nature of an emergency room, this is not always available.

Even if it is not an emergency admission, going into hospital for medical care can be particularly challenging for persons living with dementia. Hospital stays are harder for persons living with dementia and are associated with poorer outcomes than for persons who do not have cognitive impairment. Persons with cognitive impairment or dementia have longer stays in hospital and are more likely to have delirium superimposed on the pre-existing cognitive impairment. In addition, people who are admitted to hospital with cognitive impairment or dementia have higher rates of death, and one year after their hospital admission, they are more likely to be readmitted when compared with persons who are admitted to hospital who do not have cognitive impairment (Reynish et al., 2017). De Matteis et al. (2022) also found that a diagnosis of dementia was associated with increased mortality after a hospital admission, compared with older adults who did not have dementia. Factors that further increased the risk of death for persons who live with dementia after admission to hospital were infections in the blood and problems with breathing (pneumonia or respiratory failure) (De Matteis et al., 2022). It is important to note the volume of hospital beds that may be occupied by people living with dementia. In the UK, it has been found that one in four hospital beds are occupied by people living with dementia (Royal College of Psychiatrists, 2019).

The busy, noisy hospital environment, potential overcrowding, and lack of privacy can be confusing and scary, as can a new environment to navigate (Dewing & Dijk, 2016; Moyle et al., 2016). Healthcare providers might only speak with care partners and not with persons who are living with dementia, which causes them to feel uninvolved in their own care and generally unvalued (Hung et al., 2017). In fact, some research has suggested that persons with dementia who are in hospital experience care that is less than ideal regarding the preservation of dignity, privacy, and safety from rushed healthcare providers who are focused on medical care versus taking the time to provide person-centred care that takes into account the unique needs of persons living with dementia (Jurgens et al., 2012).

Attempts have been made to provide more education on dementia care to hospital staff, but generally, hospital staff report lacking education on dementia, which likely underlies many of the research reports of problems that families of persons with dementia experience in hospital settings (Dewing & Dijk, 2016).

Busy hospital staff might not know that the person in a particular hospital bed has dementia, and staff might not be aware that their patient might not understand the question they are being asked. It can help for families to ensure that the medical chart clearly identifies that the person in hospital has dementia, and it might be of benefit to provide helpful communication tips on a bedside sign. Frequently, care partners need to act as advocates for the person living with dementia when they are admitted to hospital. Encourage the healthcare team to include the person with dementia in healthcare conversations and get assent if legal consent for medical care must occur via a proxy decision-maker care partner. Care partners report that visits to hospital for people living with dementia are a particularly stressful experience, and they find they must be tireless advocates and keep a watchful eye. Some research suggests persons living with dementia who are admitted to hospital are more likely to be thirsty or hungry (or in pain) than other hospital patients because of problems with communication that can be associated with dementia (Bridges & Wilkinson, 2011). These are some of the factors underlying the reasons a person living with dementia would likely benefit from a care partner advocate during any hospital stay. In England and Wales, an audit of hospitals found that 96% of hospitals had a system in place for more flexible family visiting, enabling families to visit and the opportunity to advocate for the person living with dementia. Also, 88% of carers (and/or the person living with dementia) now receive a copy of the discharge plan (Royal College of Psychiatrists, 2019). This is a positive move forward to ensure that the family can remain involved while the person living with dementia is in hospital and is informed about the support plans when the person is discharged. The transition from hospital to return home is important to consider, as it is often a time that families and the person living with dementia experience as problematic. Guidance, such as the UK National Institute for Clinical Evidence (2015), exists to help consider how to support such transitions when the person has social care needs both before they are admitted to and when they leave hospital.

However, during the COVID-19 pandemic, the situation in hospitals rapidly changed. By the fifth audit of hospitals in England and Wales, the situation in hospitals for people living with dementia was not as positive, as no one was allowed to accompany a person admitted to hospital (Royal College of Psychiatrists, 2023). Recent qualitative interviews with care partners include stories of the person with dementia losing all personal items such as glasses and wallets with identification. It can help to plan for the eventuality of lost items even when care partners are allowed to accompany loved ones into hospital settings; send the back-up pair of glasses versus the newer pair of glasses if possible, label everything, and hope all items can be recovered if they are misplaced in the busy hospital environment.

Clearly, more needs to be done in hospital settings to improve outcomes for persons living with dementia. Recommendations that arose from a review of the scientific literature discussed placing a person at the centre of individualized care (also referred to as person-centred care), building hospitals that are accessible to all using the principles of universal design, and the need for more healthcare staff training in dementia (Røsvik & Rokstad, 2020). This review of the literature suggested that physical changes to hospitals to help people with dementia orientate to where they were and how to easily navigate to where they needed to go, and orientate to time, were particularly important. Families can facilitate orientation by bringing a very large and easy-to-read clock to the hospital room or having a large calendar with the days of the week crossed off to help orientate the person living with dementia about which day of the week it is. An orientation board that has the location of the person living with dementia (e.g. you are in hospital, you are recovering from a broken hip), the current date, and the time might also be helpful. The following includes simple

instructions on how to make an orientation board: https://www
.crossroadshospice.com/hospice-palliative-care-blog/2017/august
/16/orientation-board-activities-for-dementia-patients/#:~:text
=Caregivers%20can%20help%20by%20providing,and%20calen-
dars%20around%20the%20house.

Staff training was emphasized in the review by Røsvik and
Rokstad (2020). The Scottish National Dementia Champions
Programme focuses on training hospital staff in appropriate
dementia care and incorporates the principles of person-centred
care. An evaluation of this programme suggests that it can improve
knowledge of dementia-related care for hospital-based healthcare
staff in Scotland (Jack-Waugh et al., 2018). This programme was
recently adapted for the Canadian context (Peacock et al., 2023).
In England and Wales, a hospital audit before the COVID-19 pandemic found that 89% of hospital staff reported receiving some
dementia training (an increase of 6% from the previous audit
round), but training relevant to the grade and role of hospital staff
was still flagged as an area requiring further improvement (Royal
College of Psychiatrists, 2019). However, the audit occurring
after the height of the pandemic found that only 58% of hospitals were able to report on the dementia training that staff had
received. Hopefully, as the hospital system recovers, more jurisdictions worldwide will adopt similar training programmes for hospital staff, which will result in better care for persons living with
dementia when they are admitted to hospital.

It is also important to note that countries may lack guidelines for
the admission of people living with dementia. For example, Canada
lacks guidelines for acute care admissions or policies to better treat
persons living with dementia in hospital. In an editorial, Frank and
Molnar (2022) detail how the Canadian government's failures to
plan for hospital admissions for persons living with dementia are
short-sighted and will result in tangible risks for all Canadians who
need to use overstretched hospital resources. The cogently argued
editorial notes that an acute care plan for dementia is complex and
will require action at multiple levels. Some factors that will be

needed relate to good methods for the tracking and surveillance of issues that could impact persons with dementia in acute care and also suggest screening for cognitive impairment in all patients over 65 who present to emergency departments. A commitment to training staff and creating teams composed of medical professionals from multiple disciplines, including dementia care specialists in emergency departments will require a fundamental shift in the priorities of hospital leadership. Other recommendations include care teams involving families in care planning that is individualized, puts the needs of persons living with dementia at the core, and emphasizes non-pharmacological treatments for responsive behaviours. Finally, a recommendation to modify acute care physical spaces to be less confusing and provide much-needed stimuli that help with orientation for persons living with dementia.

Hospital care is a huge topic in and of itself. This chapter has highlighted some of the common challenges that people living with dementia and their families face, and strategies, some very simple, that can be used to help prepare for hospital appointments, as well as ideas on how it is possible to approach hospital care.

## CHAPTER 6 RESOURCES

There are suggested links to websites included in the relevant sections of this chapter. These selected resources provide additional places to find more information that may be helpful.

Alzheimer's Society. (n.d.). *Hospital care*. Retrieved March 31, 2024, from https://www.alzheimers.org.uk/sites/default/files/pdf/factsheet_hospital_care.pdf

Alzheimer's Society. (2021a). *This is me*. Retrieved March 31, 2024, from https://www.alzheimers.org.uk/sites/default/files/2020-03/this_is_me_1553.pdf

Alzheimer's Society. (2021b, December 6). *My appointments—Helping people with dementia keep track of appointments*. Retrieved March 31, 2024, from https://www.alzheimers.org.uk/get-support/publications-factsheets/my-appointments

Alzheimer's Society of B.C. (n.d.). *The dementia companion handbook*. Retrieved March 31, 2024, from https://alzheimer.ca/bc/sites/bc/files/documents/Dementia%20Companion%20Handbook_printable15.pdf

# REFERENCES

Bridges, J., & Wilkinson, C. (2011). Achieving dignity for older people with dementia in hospital. *Nursing Standard, 25*(29), 42–47 quiz 8.

Department of Health. (2019, May 27). *National dementia strategy.* https://www.gov.ie/en/publication/62d6a5-national-dementia-strategy/

Dewing, J., & Dijk, S. (2016). What is the current state of care for older people with dementia in general hospitals? A literature review. *Dementia, 15*(1), 106–124. https://doi.org/10.1177/1471301213520172

De Matteis, G., Burzo, M. L., Della Polla, D. A., Serra, A., Russo, A., Landi, F., ... & Covino, M. (2022). Outcomes and predictors of in-hospital mortality among older patients with dementia. *Journal of Clinical Medicine, 12*(1), 59.

Frank, C., & Molnar, F. (2022). Dementia care in acute care settings: Failing to plan for dementia is planning to fail. *Canadian Family Physician, 68*(1), 25–26. https://doi.org/https://doi.org/10.46747/cfp.680125

Gwernan-Jones, R., Abbott, R., Lourida, I., Rogers, M., Green, C., Ball, S., Hemsley, A., Cheeseman, D., Clare, L., Moore, D. A., Hussey, C., Coxon, G., Llewellyn, D. J., Naldrett, T., & Thompson Coon, J. (2020). The experiences of hospital staff who provide care for people living with dementia: A systematic review and synthesis of qualitative studies. *International Journal Older People Nursing, 15,* e12325. https://doi.org/10.1111/opn.12325.

Handley, M., Bunn, F., & Goodman, C. (2017). Dementia-friendly interventions to improve the care of people living with dementia admitted to hospitals: A realist review. *BMJ Open, 7,* e015257. https://doi.org/10.1136/bmjopen-2016-015257

HSE. (2021). *Vascular dementia—Causes.* HSE.Ie. https://www2.hse.ie/conditions/vascular-dementia/causes/

Hung, L., Phinney, A., Chaudhury, H., Rodney, P., Tabamo, J., & Bohl, D. (2017). "Little things matter!" Exploring the perspectives of patients with dementia about the hospital environment. *International Journal of Older People Nursing, 12*(3), e12153. https://doi.org/10.1111/opn.12153

Irish Osteoporosis Society. (2021, April 23). *About osteoporosis—Irish osteoporosis society.* https://www.irishosteoporosis.ie/information-support/about-osteoporosis/

Jack-Waugh, A., Ritchie, L., & MacRae, R. (2018). Assessing the educational impact of the dementia champions programme in Scotland: Implications for evaluating professional dementia education. *Nurse Education Today, 71,* 205–210. https://doi.org/10.1016/j.nedt.2018.09.019

Jurgens, F. J., Clissett, P., Gladman, J. R. F., & Harwood, R. H. (2012). Why are family carers of people with dementia dissatisfied with general hospital care? A qualitative study. *BMC Geriatrics, 12*(57), 1–10. https://doi.org/10.1186/1471-2318- 12-57

Manietta, C., Purwins, D., Reinhard, A., Knecht, C., & Roes, M. (2022). Characteristics of dementia-friendly hospitals: An integrative review. *BMC Geriatr, 22*, 468. https://doi.org/10.1186/s12877-022-03103-6

Moyle, W., Bramble, M., Bauer, M., Smyth, W., & Beattie, E. (2016). 'They rush you and push you too much... and you can't really get any good response off them': A qualitative examination of family involvement in care of people with dementia in acute care. *Australasian Journal on Ageing, 35*(2), E30–E34. https://doi.org/10.1111/ajag.12251

NICE. (2021). *NICEimpact dementia: Hospital care.* National Institute for Health and Care Excellence. https://www.nice.org.uk/about/what-we-do/into-practice/measuring-the-use-of-nice-guidance/impact-of-our-guidance/niceimpact-dementia/ch3-hospital-care

Peacock, S., Bayly, M., Fletcher-Hildebrand, S., Gibson, K., MacRae, R., Jack-Waugh, A., Haase, K., Bally, J., Duggleby, W., Hall, S., Holtslander, L., McAiney, C., Michael, J., Morgan, D., O'Connell, M.E., Ploeg, J., Rohatinsky, N., Thompson, G., & Vedel, I. (2023). Championing dementia education: Adapting an effective scottish dementia education program for canadian acute health care providers. *Canadian Journal on Aging/La Revue canadienne du vieillissement, 42*(1), 165–176.

Reynish, E. L., Hapca, S. M., De Souza, N., Cvoro, V., Donnan, P. T., Guthrie, B. (2017). Epidemiology and outcomes of people with dementia, delirium, and unspecified cognitive impairment in the general hospital: Prospective cohort study of 10,014 admissions. *BMC Medicine, 15*, 140. https://doi.org/10.1186/s12916-017-0899-0

Røsvik, J., & Rokstad, A. M. M. (2020). What are the needs of people with dementia in acute hospital settings, and what interventions are made to meet these needs? A systematic integrative review of the literature. *BMC health services research, 20*, 1–20.

Royal College of Psychiatrists. (2019). *National audit of dementia care in general hospitals 2018–2019: Round four audit report.* Royal College of Psychiatrists https://www.hqip.org.uk/wp-content/uploads/2019/07/ref-113-national-audit-of-dementia-round-4-report-final-online-v4.pdf

Royal College of Psychiatrists. (2023). *National audit of dementia care in general hospitals 2022–23: Round 5 audit local report.* Healthcare Quality Improvement Partnership. Available from: www.nationalauditofdementia.org.uk

The Butterfly Scheme. (2016). *The butterfly scheme has gone international!* https://butterflyscheme.org.uk/september-2016/

# Part 3

# 7

## HOW DO WE PLAN A MOVE TO LONG-STAY CARE?

### HOW DO YOU EVALUATE IF CARE NEEDS EXCEED WHAT YOU CAN OFFER SAFELY AT HOME?

One of the most challenging worries that is shared by families and persons living with dementia is 'what to do when care needs exceed what can be safely offered at home'. Frequently, the family member living with dementia has communicated on multiple occasions (likely over several years preceding the diagnosis of dementia) their preference to remain in their own home and to avoid an admission to residential or long-term care. Research suggests that most ageing people express a desire to age at home, but a multitude of factors influence preferences to age at home (Roy et al., 2018). Persons living with dementia might change their views on ageing at home from those they might have expressed prior to the onset of dementia. In fact, research suggests that the preferences of persons with dementia to receive in-home care to meet their daily needs change as care needs become more extensive; when care needs become extensive, most persons with dementia who were asked their preferences stated that they would prefer residential care (Lehnert et al., 2019). Why do the preferences of persons living with dementia for in-home and residential care change as care needs increase? A review of the available research reveals

DOI: 10.4324/9781003457138-10

that the top concern for most people diagnosed with dementia is the quality of life of their care partners, and, further, persons with dementia worry about being perceived as a burden by their care partners (Wehrmann et al., 2021). These findings help us to generate several hypotheses of the psychological mechanisms that underlie a change in preference from in-home to residential care: as care needs increase, persons with dementia perceive care partner burden to increase and worry about declines in their care partner's quality of life, which likely influence their preferences for residential care.

Many families experience a sense of angst and uncertainty regarding making decisions about placement in long-term care, with the most pressing decision being the timing of admission to long-term care. In many jurisdictions, there is a greater need for long-term care beds than are available, and consequently, the decision regarding admission to long-term care is not made by persons living with dementia or their families. Commonly, there is a formal service that acts as a gatekeeper regarding eligibility for long-term care admission based on the care needs of the person living with dementia. In circumstances where eligibility for long-term care is dependent on a gatekeeper's assessment of the level of care needs, families can refuse long-term care admission if offered, but frequently families cannot decide to admit a person living with dementia to long-term care if their care needs are not sufficiently high to make persons with dementia eligible for long-term care. It is important to stress that the processes for long-term care admission and eligibility vary greatly by region. However, worldwide projections suggest that there will continue to be more need for long-term care beds than are available. Some families' experiences with long-term care admission decisions are clarified by the gatekeeping-type assessment, and a healthcare professional makes it clear to families that keeping their loved one at home is no longer safe or sufficient for quality care. Some families find hearing an outsider's assessment of the care situation a relief – the decision they have been stressing about for months or even years is no longer theirs to make, and the healthcare professional's assessment provides something akin to permission that relieves a sense of personal guilt at making a decision for long-term care admission. However, some families do not wish to admit their loved one to long-term care even after a healthcare professional suggests that it is likely the safest and most appropriate option; the reasons for this vary widely but can include a strong sense of personal responsibility for care (reflecting strong culturally bound core values for many persons), concerns about the cost of long-term care, and concerns about the quality of long-term care.

It is clear that long-term care can be the most appropriate level of care for persons living with dementia under several circumstances, including safety and care partner exhaustion. A review of the research by Teng et al. (2020) revealed that some of the safety needs that precipitate a need for long-term care admission include avoiding injury for those living with dementia who are medically frail, which can include people who have a high risk of falls or a high risk of personal injury from falling. Another safety issue that can be a strong factor in suggesting that long-term care is the most appropriate living situation for a person living with dementia is concerns about wandering or getting lost that can put them at high risk of personal injury. On occasion, the risk of personal injury is a risk for care partners, and this situation can suggest that long-term care is the most appropriate living situation for a person living with dementia. If, for example, persons living with dementia experience extreme confusion, there have been reports of physical aggression causing bodily harm to those who are providing care. Thankfully, these reports do not reflect the typical experience of many care partners, but when it does occur, it is extremely distressing for those in a caregiving role, whether they are family care partners or formal caregivers who are healthcare providers. Care needs that exceed the capacity of the caregiving team are another reason that long-term care is most appropriate to meet the needs of the person living with dementia – whether that is a solo care partner who has caregiving duties 24 hours a day, seven days a week, or a team involved in caregiving, which can include family care partners receiving in-home formal care support. Reasons for care partner exhaustion can include the long duration of providing a high level of care (e.g. the need to clean up after bowel incontinence) and chronic sleep disturbance. Care partners are most able to provide appropriate care when they get an opportunity to rest and recuperate, and in many jurisdictions, this can involve formal respite care or informal support from an extended family or friend network to provide the primary care partner with a break to catch up on sleep and engage in some much-needed self-care. Being a care partner is not a sprint, it is a marathon, and running as fast as one would for a sprint without pacing means that one would make completing a marathon impossible.

Using respite care, defined here as 'a defined time for an alternate care arrangement for the person living with dementia who needs daily and nightly care', can help care partners complete the marathon. The research literature suggests that, under certain circumstances, some care partners can benefit from respite care, but numerous factors impact the satisfaction of care partners with respite care, including the perceived quality of the respite care, whether respite care actually provides care partners with relief from caregiving duties, and whether they feel secure about the comfort and safety of the person living with dementia (Neville et al., 2015).

## HOW DO YOU LEARN TO LIVE WITH RISK?

Chapter 3 discussed thinking about risk when engaging in discussions regarding advance care planning. Ideally, all family members agree in these discussions, and ideally, these discussions empower the person living with dementia to have their voice, preferences, and wishes for the future heard by all family members. Some family members, who are highly risk-averse, have views that come from a place of caring for the person living with dementia, but to avoid all risk takes away the autonomy, agency, and empowerment of the person living with dementia. If, for example, problems with wayfinding create a risk of getting lost or injured, a reasonable and highly risk-averse approach would be to remove all possibility that the person with dementia could get lost. However, to do this would involve restricting the movement of the person living with dementia by locking them in a secure location; indeed, many long-term care placements are secure and restrict the ability of the person with dementia to exercise agency in their movements outside the secure unit. Removal of risk is almost invariably accompanied by a loss of autonomy and agency for the person living with dementia, underscoring the importance of empowering the person living with dementia to engage in advance care planning discussions regarding their views on risk and preferences for balancing risk and autonomy when their care needs progress and their ability to communicate their preferences and engage in care planning diminishes.

Families who understand that the only way to remove risk comes at the cost of autonomy for the person living with dementia can rationalize living with a level of risk, and they can use this rationalization to manage their anxiety and fears for their loved one living with dementia. To live with risk requires care partners to holistically consider the quality of life of the person with dementia. This includes a consideration of the fundamental human rights of the person living with dementia, including dignity, autonomy, and self-determination. The World Health Organization (WHO) has an excellent resource on human rights for persons living with dementia (WHO, 2015).

https://www.ohchr.org/sites/default/files/Documents/Issues/OlderPersons/Dementia/ThematicBrief.pdf

## HOW SHOULD DECISIONS REGARDING LONG-TERM CARE BE APPROACHED WHEN THERE IS FAMILY DISAGREEMENT?

A frequent source of disagreement for families of persons living with dementia can be distilled as different views on risk tolerance, which can lead to disagreements about whether long-term care is the most appropriate living situation for their loved one with dementia. It would be ideal if discussions with all family members privileged the preferences expressed by the person with dementia. Many conversations held when engaging in advance care planning do not take on board the person living with dementia's preferences, rather they centre around the preferences of the family members. Ideally those provided with the responsibility for proxy decision-making in the event of the diminished capacity of the person with dementia held similar views on risk versus autonomy as the person with dementia and similar values regarding the quality of life of the person with dementia. Even in an ideal situation such as the one described, invariably there are situations that were not discussed during the advance care planning, and proxy decision-makers must infer what the person living with dementia would prefer regarding their care, providing multiple possibilities for family disagreements. Recent research suggests that care partners who experience disagreements in how best to provide care for their loved one with dementia are more likely to report symptoms of depression and anxiety, and high levels of perceived caregiver burden (Xu et al., 2021). Proxy decision-makers who disagree regarding the most appropriate course of action for caring for the person living with dementia can come to an impasse and might need legal recourse to identify a sole proxy decision-maker. This is, hopefully, the last resort. Many care partners experience disagreements regarding the best care for the person living with dementia that are not extreme enough to require legal recourse, but any form of disagreement can rip a family apart. The stress of having contrary views on the best care for the person living with dementia is added to pre-existing family relationship dynamics, which can be complicated and rife with unspoken conflict that contributes to an escalation in conflict. In general, de-escalation techniques can help during the most stressful phase of a conflict. Hostility exacerbates hostility and calm communication helps to de-escalate conflict. If you are unable to remain calm, it might be best to re-attempt the conversation at a later time.

Part of the reason why disagreements about the care for the person with dementia are so stressful for care partners is that no one can predict the best course of action with absolute certainty. Recall that a reduction in risk comes at the cost of the quality of life and could violate the human rights of the person living with dementia. No decision here is an easy decision, and there is no litmus test to tell anyone involved which decision is the right one at any given time. Living with uncertainty is psychologically distressing for most people. Reaching out to formal care supports, particularly those that provide reassurance that the care provided is the best care possible given the circumstances, can be helpful. Seeking support from others who have been in similar situations can also be helpful, such as through a support group.

Few people know how to have a conversation in the context of conflict. A myriad of online resources provide advice on how to have a conversation, and even master classes are available. At the core, begin by respectfully asking the person with whom you need to have a conversation if this is a good time to talk. Speak about what you feel you need to speak about, and listen to the response. Ideally, rephrase what you think you understand your counterpart is trying to say – this active listening strategy helps to make the person you are speaking with feel heard and has the added benefit of ensuring you actually understand what they are telling you. Avoid attacks and speak about how you feel or how the situation impacts you emotionally. If you spend more time listening and understanding than you do speaking, you are more likely to successfully communicate understanding – even if you still disagree. People are more likely to stay stuck in their opinion when they feel unheard and their viewpoint is not understood. Understanding is not agreeing. If you both communicate that your common ground is the wish to care as best as possible for the person living with dementia, it could help de-escalate conflict. Seeking support as a family to navigate difficult conversations with the assistance of a therapist or mediator could also help to mitigate conflict. Given how high the stakes are, agreeing to disagree is not likely possible, and avoiding a difficult conversation about disagreements in care plans is not advisable.

Carmel reflects on her experiences:

This was something that had come up on a number of occasions – Mum first went to a care home in 2010 because I was taking my Dad from the hospital to my home to die. He had received a very late diagnosis of colon cancer, and his wish was to die at home.

My house was the easiest to accommodate two hospital beds and all the activities that would ensue.

One of my sisters and I dropped Mum at the care home – it really felt overcrowded; it was a community facility for respite for people with dementia. Mum did not want to stay; I was in shock and unable to think, so I left her – I regret this still. When I collected her again, she was very sad and confused.

We got home, and we cared for Dad for 12 days and nights with the help of the community palliative care provided by the Galway hospice. The staff had to be transported daily by the army due to horrendous weather conditions that December (2010) Galway Hospice (2024).

I did use residential care for respite in 2011 and 2012, but I always brought Mum to see it first. Even then, the actual lived experience during the stay was not what we expected.

I now advocate for respite to be provided in the home residence rather than moving the person and causing total confusion.

One of my main concerns about residential care is the use of antipsychotic drugs. They are far too prevalent in care facilities.

A research project (Walsh et al., 2017) regarding the use of antipsychotics in care homes is very interesting and also shows that their use is not the sole solution. Once again, person-centred care is the key to our well-being.

## THINGS HAVE BECOME TOO MUCH TO COPE WITH AT HOME. HOW DO WE MAKE THE DECISION TO LOOK FOR LONG-STAY SUPPORT?

The decision to place a person with dementia in institutional care is a difficult one for family care partners. This reflects the challenges more broadly reported in the research literature around older adults moving to long-term care (Egan et al., 2023). This difficulty may be resolved by a crisis situation where the decision is 'made' by circumstances. For example, it may be that the health of the care partner deteriorates and they are unable to continue providing care for the person living with dementia as they now need support and care to meet their own needs. Or it may be that the emotional trauma, including lack of sleep due to nighttime care support required, of caregiving over a sustained time may become too much and may result in a decision to explore the options of moving the person to a care setting. Or it could be that providing adequate care and support, such as pain relief and other treatments, becomes increasingly difficult for the care partner to achieve. The help of care professionals may be required on a 24-hour basis that cannot be provided in the person's own home, no matter how much creativity is explored to find ways to provide that care in the home of the person living with dementia. The circumstances surrounding the decision to make the transition from home to institution are likely to have an impact on the transition period and longer-term success, or difficulties with the transition. If the person can be involved in the decision-making process, the experience tends to be more positive; however, joint decision-making is not always a reality for the older adult (O'Neill et al., 2020).

Family members often discuss the challenges of finding a suitable care home for the person living with dementia and what they need to look for in a setting. The decision is delayed, or an application is not submitted as the care partner and the person living with dementia adjust to the knowledge of the changes that a move to a care setting will have for each individual and their relationship.

Family members have many questions when they start to consider a care home placement: How might that setting work in practice to visit the person living with dementia? Does the setting have activities and opportunities to participate in enjoyable and meaningful pursuits for the person living with dementia? Important questions for the care partner to consider when looking at care homes relate to the physical setting, its location in relation to the person's home, if there is a single room on a floor that is more accessible, if the room has a view, the staffing levels, the standard of food, if family members are welcome to visit, if there are daily activities that the person living with dementia may enjoy (or not). Family members often find it difficult to reconcile their needs and the needs of the person living with dementia as they move towards making a decision that the person living with dementia will move into long-term care.

Research also provides evidence that care partners often struggle with feelings of guilt at no longer being able to support the person living with dementia in their own home. They may also struggle with the change in their role from primary care partner to visiting a family member at the care home. This is particularly true for spousal care partners who have struggled to continue to provide care at home leading up to the transition to long-term care. It is important for family members to recognize that they have been providing support and care to the best of their ability for as long as possible. It is also important to consider whether the homes being appraised include the family as much as possible in the care of their relative and how they discuss issues in a way that promotes open and honest communication between the family members and care home staff.

It is not only care partners who find the move to long-term care difficult. The person living with dementia might also experience feelings of loss and bereavement or difficulties associated with finding themselves in a communal living environment where they no longer have as much choice and independence over their day-to-day life. As the person living with dementia adjusts to living in the care home, they may feel unease at strangers (the care staff) invading their personal space, providing personal care, or simply not recognizing new faces as shifts change and new staff come on duty. This means that the transition to long-term care can be challenging for both the person living with dementia and their care partner (Sury et al., 2013). In their review, Groenvynck et al. (2022) found that different supports can help the transition for everyone, including education, relationships/communication, improving emotional well-being, personalized care, continuity of care, support provision, and ad hoc counselling. This means that it is possible to make the transition less difficult with the right kinds of support and planning (before a crisis arises).

# WHAT ARE THE THINGS TO LOOK FOR IN A CARE HOME/LONG-STAY CARE SETTING?

## CARE HOME/LONG-TERM CARE TRANSITION

The time has arrived to consider a transition to a care home or nursing home. It is a time when, as a care partner, the person with the diagnosis, or the health professional making the recommendation, you may be feeling many emotions over having to do this, and you may have many questions and concerns. It is at this point in the journey with dementia when the spouse or care partner may begin to make decisions about and for their loved one.

Phyllis reflects on this issue from a personal standpoint:

Hopefully, you have had a chance to discuss and plan for this ahead of time. Usually, by the time this stage happens, the person living with dementia has a hard time understanding or giving input. They may not be able to express their thoughts or wishes. A prior discussion with them would help you to know what they think and want at this stage. Speaking from experience, I discussed this in detail with my family. We talked about which homes in our area I would like to go to and what I wanted to happen surrounding my care. We even put together a guide of my likes and dislikes, my wishes, and things that are important for the new carers to know. I will go into more details as we move through this chapter.

To look at the timing around this decision, we need to answer the questions: When is the right time? Is it the right time? How do we know when it's time? Let me say that I don't think there is ever a set or right time because the timing depends on so many other factors. I think first we have to look at the person living with dementia and ask ourselves a few questions: Are they coping? Are they able to care for themselves? Are they having to rely on others for their personal care? Are they ready? Am I giving up all my time in order to help them? Some other big questions could be about yourself as a care partner or a spouse: Are you losing yourself caring for them? Are you able to do things you want to do? Are you losing your friends and family and loved ones because all your time is spent caring for that other person?

For persons living with young-onset Alzheimer's, like me, the questions may include: Are they too young to go into a nursing home? How will they fit in? Some of the things you may have to consider when you are in this situation, especially with young-onset dementia, are the family dynamics. You may still be working, you may still have a young family, you may be caring for elderly parents. All these things factor in when making this decision. You may worry about how others see you and what they think of you. You may feel like a failure, like you are giving up; but let me remind you, no one but you is walking this journey. Only you know what's happening, how you are feeling, and how the person with dementia is truly doing. Unless someone else is living and dealing with this, they truly don't know; they only see glimpses of what's happening. I would like to take a moment to remind you that you truly are not going through this alone. There is help out there and sometimes it's best to talk to someone. Your family doctor can help, or counsellors are available through the Alzheimer Society. Maybe you can talk to others who have already gone through this.

Another thing to consider is the process of doing this. This process is not easy as you have to fill out paperwork and you have to make decisions regarding which nursing home to choose. You may feel that the time is right, and the time is now, but the lengthy time it takes to process the paperwork may cause delays. The other factor that is key here is, depending on the area you live in, there may be a long waiting list for a nursing home, which will delay placement of your loved one. If this happens, how are you going to cope or manage during the waiting period? These are questions that I ask myself as I think through how I might prepare for this final transition if it is needed.

## HOW CAN THE FAMILY STAY INVOLVED WHEN THE PERSON MOVES INTO LONG-STAY CARE?

Of course, circumstances may change, and a loved one might have to move to long-term care. We can never guarantee that circumstances will not change. So, for this reason, and to ensure your loved one is going to get the best care possible and have some input into their future, it would be prudent to explore some possibilities in your area. I would love to see a residential facility in all communities; it should be an integral part. It would be such a comfort to individuals and family members to know that such a place exists if the need arises to use the facilities.

Families can try to organize a plan for visiting, taking their loved one out, or whatever is needed and suits them. Some like to visit at mealtimes and sit with their loved one, which helps ensure they eat and have liquids. Medication may need to be given at a certain time, and this, again, may be a responsibility that a family member would like to oversee. Having input like this can sometimes help the family member who is perhaps feeling guilty and feels they have let down their loved one.

Many people love visiting neighbours and friends in care homes as they feel it is less pressure and there are more distractions on which to comment. With modern technology, it is now very convenient for people to connect via iPhone, Zoom, and social media, giving those who have moved further away an opportunity to keep in regular contact with their loved ones.

It is also an opportunity to still share interests like gardening – encourage a polytunnel, raised beds, potted plants, and the produce can then be used in the kitchen (Engaging Dementia, 2024).

Sensory gardens are very therapeutic not only for a person with a dementia diagnosis but also for all the residents, staff, and visitors (Centre for Sustainable Healthcare, n.d.). It is a beautiful way to interact and also opens up opportunities for intergenerational projects. A sensory garden stimulates the five senses: sight, smell, hearing, touch, and taste. The experience is not just about the planting; it takes in the pathway, a water feature, and the sound of flowing water. It helps with agitation, feelings of uselessness, isolation, value, and inclusion, as it promotes being part of a team.

## HOW CAN YOU COMMUNICATE WITH THE LONG-TERM CARE HOME AND BE AN ADVOCATE?

When we think of this question, some people can actually do this naturally without having to think about it, but others may struggle.

People truly only want what is best for their loved one; they may feel overwhelmed when their loved one goes into care. This is usually brought on by feelings of inadequacy, failure, and loss of control. In their discussion about adult daughters advocating for their parent when the parent is in a care setting, Legault and Ducharme (2009) demonstrate that this role evolves over time. Although discussing adult daughters' experiences, this process of an evolving advocacy role is one that all care partners may experience, regardless of the relationship to the person living with dementia.

When a loved one goes into care, communication is key. Let's first consider the feelings that everyone may be dealing with, because if we don't address this issue, we may never be able to move forward and become the support and advocate that the person living with dementia needs. It is at this time that care partners may be a ball of emotions; after providing support and care, it is common to be exhausted and both physically and mentally drained. There are numerous reasons for this, depending on each personal situation: being an only child, primary care partner, having or not having power of attorney for personal care, just to list a few. There will be times when continuing to be involved in the care and support of the person living with dementia is challenging. The global COVID-19 pandemic is a stark reminder of this, when the challenges family members faced were compounded by not being able to visit their family member (Mitchell et al., 2022).

One of the best things to do is to understand that feelings are to be expected; what is 'normal' varies for each individual. Some people don't realize how much stress they have been under and are exhausted. Care partners may feel a sense of relief, loss of control over the care, or there may be numbness, a sense of feeling nothing at all. We ask ourselves, what happens now? This is the time when it is important for the care partner to take some time for themselves, knowing that someone else is caring for their loved one. That is not always easy! But to enable time to recover from caregiving, it is important to remember that the staff is trained in what they do, and that opportunities to visit and be involved in ongoing support will be available. Depending on the situation, it is likely that prior to admission various facilities were visited and a selection was made (unless a crisis situation has led to no choice of location), but whatever the situation, it is important that the paperwork is completed and that it includes as much information as possible about the person living with dementia to assist staff in providing the best possible care.

We suggest that in the early days of settling in, it can be helpful to visit often and get to know the staff. Help by informing them about the preferences and needs of the person living with dementia, what they like, who they are, and how they did things. The more they know about the person living with dementia, the better, as this can help care staff to become connected and engaged with them. It is, of course, a balancing act of sharing information while not being seen as 'taking over' or 'distrusting' staff. Relationship building between staff and family is key to advocating for the person living with dementia and ensuring that their best interests can be met.

## CHAPTER 7 RESOURCES

We have collated a selection of resources that provide clear information about issues that are important to consider when thinking about a care home or long-term care. These may be helpful when looking into a care home in the place where one lives.

Alzheimer's Association (US). (2023). *Choosing a residential care community.* Retrieved March 31, 2024, from https://www.alz.org/media/documents/ alzheimers-dementia-choosing-residential-care-ts.pdf

Alzheimer's Association (US). (2022). *Home safety checklist.* Retrieved March 31, 2024, from https://www.alz.org/media/documents/alzheimers -dementia-home-safety-checklist-ts.pdf

Alzheimer Society of Canada. (2018). *Dementia and living alone.* Retrieved March 31, 2024, from https://archive.alzheimer.ca/sites/default/files /bc/dementia-and-living-alone%20(feb%202018)_0.pdf

Armstrong, P., & Lowndes, R. (2018). *Negotiating tensions in long-term residential care: Ideas worth sharing.* Canadian Center for Policy Alternatives. Retrieved March 31, 2024, from https://policyalternatives.ca/sites/default /files/uploads/publications/National%20Office/2018/05/Negotiating %20Tensions.pdf

Alzheimer Society of Canada. (2022). *Considering the move to a long-term care home.* Retrieved March 31, 2024, from https://alzheimer.ca/sites/default /files/documents/Long-term-care-1-Considering-the-move-Alzheimer -Society.pdf

Alzheimer's Society (UK). (n.d). How do you know if someone needs to move into a care home? Retrieved March 31, 2024, from https:// www.alzheimers.org.uk/get-support/help-dementia-care/care-homes -decision

Berg, V. (2023). *When should someone with dementia move into a care home?* Care Home UK. Retrieved March 31, 2024, from https://www.carehome.co.uk /advice/when-should-someone-with-dementia-move-into-a-care-home

Dementia UK. (2022). *Considering a care home for a person with dementia.* Dementia UK. Retrieved March 31, 2024, from https://www.dementiauk .org/wp-content/uploads/2023/07/dementia-uk-considering-care-home .pdf

Government of British Columbia. (2021). *Planning for your care needs: Considerations in selecting a long-term care home.* Retrieved March 31, 2024, from https://www2.gov.bc.ca/assets/gov/health/accessing-health-care/ finding-assisted-living-residential-care-facilities/residential-care-facilities/ planning-for-your-care-needs-2021.pdf

NHS England. (2022). *Dementia and care homes.* Retrieved March 31, 2024, from https://www.nhs.uk/conditions/dementia/care-and-support/care -homes/#:~:text=Deciding%20to%20move%20into%20a%20care%20home &text=But%20the%20person%20with%20dementia,it's%20in%20their%20 best%20interests

# REFERENCES

Centre for Sustainable Healthcare. (n.d.). Sensory and dementia gardens. *NHS Forest.* Retrieved March 28, 2024, from https://nhsforest.org/green -your-site/sensory-and-dementia-gardens/

*Community Palliative Care.* (2024). Galway Hospice Foundation. https:// galwayhospice.ie/hospice-care/community-palliative-care/

Egan, C., Naughton, C., Caples, M., & Mulcahy, H. (2023). Shared decision-making with adults transitioning to long-term care: A scoping review. *International Journal of Older People Nursing, 18*(1), e12518. https://doi.org /10.1111/opn.12518

Engaging Dementia. (2024). Make your garden dementia friendly. *Engaging Dementia.* https://engagingdementia.ie/what-we-do/activity-resources/ make-your-garden-dementia-friendly/

Groenvynck, L., Fakha, A., de Boer, B., Hamers, J. P. H., van Achterberg, T., van Rossum, E., & Verbeek, H. (2022). Interventions to improve the transition from home to a nursing home: A scoping review. *The Gerontologist, 62*(7), e369–e383. https://doi.org/10.1093/geront/gnab036

Hanssen, I., Mkhonto, F. M., Øieren, H., Sengane, M. L., Sørensen, A. L., & Tran, P. T. M. (2022). Pre-decision regret before transition of dependents with severe dementia to long-term care. *Nursing Ethics, 29*(2), 344–355. https://doi.org/10.1177/09697330211015339

Larsen, L. S., Blix, B. H., & Hamran, T. (2020). Family caregivers' involvement in decision-making processes regarding admission of persons with dementia to nursing homes. *Dementia,19*(6), 2038–2055. https://doi.org/10.1177/1471301218814641

Lehnert, T., Heuchert, M. A. X., Hussain, K., & Koenig, H. H. (2019). Stated preferences for long-term care: A literature review. *Ageing & Society, 39*(9), 1873–1913.

Legault, A., & Ducharme, F. (2009). Advocating for a parent with dementia in a long-term care facility: The process experienced by daughters. *Journal of Family Nursing, 15*(2), 198–219. https://doi.org/10.1177/1074840709332929

Mitchell, L. L., Albers, E. A., Birkeland, R. W., Peterson, C. M., Stabler, H., Horn, B., Cha, J., Drake, A., & Gaugler, J. E. (2022). Caring for a relative with dementia in long-term care during COVID-19. *Journal American Medical Directors Association, 23*(3), 428–433.e1. https://doi.org/10.1016/j.jamda.2021.11.026

Neville, C., Beattie, E., Fielding, E., & MacAndrew, M. (2015). Literature review: Use of respite by carers of people with dementia. *Health & Social Care in the Community, 23*(1), 51–63

O'Neill, M., Ryan, A., Tracey, A., & Laird, L. (2020). "You're at their mercy": Older peoples' experiences of moving from home to a care home: A grounded theory study. *International Journal of Older People Nursing, 15*(2), 1–14. https://doi.org/10.1111/opn.12305

Roy, N., Dubé, R., Després, C., Freitas, A., & Légaré, F. (2018). Choosing between staying at home or moving: A systematic review of factors influencing housing decisions among frail older adults. *PloS one, 13*(1), e0189266.

Schulz, R., Belle, S. H., Czaja, S. J., McGinnis, K. A., Stevens, A., & Zhang, S. (2004). Long-term care placement of dementia patients and caregiver health and well-being. *JAMA, 292*(8), 961–967. https://doi.org/10.1001/jama.292.8.961

Sury, L., Burns, K., & Brodaty, H. (2013). Moving in: Adjustment of people living with dementia going into a nursing home and their families. *International Psychogeriatrics, 25*(6), 867–876. https://doi.org/10.1017/S1041610213000057

Teng, C., Loy, C. T., Sellars, M., Pond, D., Latt, M. D., Waite, L. M., ... & Tong, A. (2020). Making decisions about long-term institutional care placement among people with dementia and their caregivers: Systematic review of qualitative studies. *The Gerontologist*, *60*(4), e329–e346.

Walsh, K. A., Dennehy, R., Sinnott, C., Browne, J., Byrne, S., McSharry, J., Coughlan, E., & Timmons, S. (2017). Influences on decision-making regarding antipsychotic prescribing in nursing home residents with dementia: A systematic review and synthesis of qualitative evidence. *Journal of the American Medical Directors Association*, *18*(10), 897.e1–897.e12. https://doi.org/10.1016/j.jamda.2017.06.032

Wehrmann, H., Michalowsky, B., Lepper, S., Mohr, W., Raedke, A., & Hoffmann, W. (2021). Priorities and preferences of people living with dementia or cognitive impairment–a systematic review. *Patient Preference and Adherence*, *15*, 2793–2807.

WHO. (2015). *Ensuring a human rights-based approach for people living with dementia.* https://www.ohchr.org/sites/default/files/Documents/Issues/OlderPersons/Dementia/ThematicBrief.pdf

Xu, J., Liu, P. J., & Beach, S. (2021). Multiple caregivers, many minds: Family discord and caregiver outcomes. *The Gerontologist*, *61*(5), 661–669.

# 8

---

# HOW DO WE DEAL
# WITH END-OF-LIFE AND
# PALLIATIVE CARE?

In 2004, Weafer et al. found that most older people want to stay
and die in their own home, but it is estimated that only 20% actually get to experience this, as the majority of older people die
in long-stay care or acute settings (Irish Hospice Foundation &
McKeown, 2014).

## WHAT IS END-OF-LIFE CARE OR
## PALLIATIVE CARE?

The term 'end-of-life care' is generally applied to those who are
approaching death, with a key goal to make the person comfortable and to attend to their needs and wishes as the end of their
life approaches. One of the key aspects of such an approach is that
it recognizes that much can still be done, even when a cure is
no longer an option (Janssens, 2004). End-of-life care, as a subject, was slow to appear in the dementia care literature. This led
to the quality of end-of-life care being overlooked in dementia
care for many years. As has been highlighted, when it was discussed in the early days, it was perceived as a taboo area (Cox &
Watchman, 2004). Accessible, good practice guides emerged (e.g.
Kelly & Innes, 2010; Davies & Iliffe, 2020) primarily aimed at

DOI: 10.4324/9781003457138-11

health and social care professionals. However, end of life remains a critical phase in the lives of people with dementia, their families, and those who care for them, and there is only one chance to get it right. One definition of end-of-life care proposed by Ross et al. (2000) encompasses a sensitive, individually focused, compassionate, and supportive approach to living with, or dying from, progressive or chronic life-threatening conditions in older people. The importance of end-of-life and palliative care has been advocated by the World Health Organization (1990) as an area requiring improvement for many years. Yet, in 2020, the WHO estimated that only 14% of those who require palliative care actually receive this form of support. Overall, research demonstrates that palliative care remains woefully inadequate (Horton, 2018). The United Nations (UN) Committee on Economic Social and Cultural Rights acknowledged palliative care as a component of the right to health in August 2000. The move towards realizing this in practice has been slow in general, and for people living with dementia in particular (Antonacci et al., 2020; Pandpazir & Tajari, 2019). However, where it does exist, the standard of care provided is high. The challenge is that it is not available to everyone, and those with dementia are at particular risk of receiving low-quality end-of-life care (Miele et al., 2022). The consequence of not receiving end-of-life care support takes its toll on family members. For example, in a US study, the year before the death of the person living with dementia, 59% of care partners reported feeling 'on duty' 24 hours a day, and 72% reported feeling relief when the person died (Schulz et al., 2003).

End-of-life care is also a term used instead of palliative care for people with a terminal disease other than cancer, because palliative care is commonly associated with people living with cancer. End-of-life care is a broader term and indicates that the end of life may be very close. It can often appear that there is little awareness or knowledge in the community about what end-of-life care means. The term 'end-of-life care' is often used interchangeably with 'palliative care', but palliative care is frequently seen in the context of hospice-based care and dying, mainly from cancer. Many countries have established policies and bodies to guide the implementation of palliative care. For example, in 2009, the Irish Hospice Foundation, along with the Health Service Executive and the Irish College of General Practitioners, established the Primary Care Palliative Care Steering Committee (Irish Hospice Foundation, 2020). The main aim of the initial phase of the work programme was to identify palliative care initiatives that would support, advise, and educate primary care teams to support and manage the care of those with advancing progressive diseases who live in their communities.

The All Ireland Institute of Hospice and Palliative Care (AIIHPC) was formally established in October 2010. It came about after a successful bid by consortium members to secure funding for the organization. Consortium members and their organizations are experts in palliative care service planning and delivery, education and training, research, and policy analysis. The aim of AIIHPC is to promote the public and professional voice of hospice and palliative care. The institute encourages debate, facilitates the promotion of palliative care issues among national policymakers (both in Northern Ireland and the Republic of Ireland), and works effectively with international partners to integrate palliative care issues into national and international healthcare agendas. Voices4Care (https://aiihpc.org/voices4care/) is an initiative of the All Ireland Institute of Hospice and Palliative Care, aiming to involve people receiving palliative care (service users), carers, and the wider community in their work. The institute is consistently working on a public awareness campaign for end-of-life care to become an integrated part of its work. The campaign builds awareness and understanding of palliative care among the general public. This is an important example to consider as the global population is ageing and will challenge the economic sustainability of the care of older people in residential care. Therefore, it is imperative that we encourage and support end-of-life care in our communities.

Primary care workers, including general practitioners, require training around what end-of-life care means and their role in administering it to their patients living with dementia. (Sideman et al., 2023). At present, the best-performing services are the hospice home care teams, but these are not available to all patients needing end-of-life care. Especially if a person lives in a rural area, these essential services are non-existent. Unfortunately, this is why, at the end of life, people are sent from their homes and residential care homes to a hospital. More families want their loved ones to remain at home, where the environment would hopefully be less stressful, more secure, and familiar to their loved ones. To facilitate this, access to medical care and pain control is essential. Most fear that they will not be in a position to control the pain; they want respect shown at all times and the dignity of their loved one to always be respected. Access to an interdisciplinary team, i.e. dietician, occupational therapist, and speech therapist, is very important. The occupational therapist provides advice on the chairs, cushions, and equipment needed; the dietician is essential for nutritional advice; and the speech therapist can monitor in case of loss of ability to swallow. A caseworker to liaise with all the supports and services on their behalf would make such a difference to a family.

The importance of the role of allied health professionals (AHP) in supporting people living with dementia is being acknowledged, and different approaches and frameworks have been developed. For example, the allied healthcare approach is relatively new in Scotland, and an allied health professionals dementia framework has been developed for Wales (Alzheimer Scotland, 2024; Welsh Government, 2022). The Scottish model comprises five key areas that have been identified as areas where allied health professionals can make a positive difference to people living with dementia, including supporting families and carers as equal partners, enhancing daily living, adapting everyday environments, maximizing psychological well-being, and maximizing physical well-being. Each of these domains needs to be considered holistically and as part of an allied healthcare professional approach to supporting people living with dementia. This approach is working well in Scotland, and Ireland is working to integrate the concept into the awareness of health and social care professionals from early career. The Welsh framework recognizes the strengths-based approach of AHPs and is committed to an enabling, person-centred, and holistic approach to delivering care, support, and interventions that is underpinned by kindness and understanding (Welsh Government, 2022, p. 13).

If medical professionals are trained in a team network, then results will be far more positive. Palliative care can span various time frames, and it is important to factor in respite for the family members. It is also important to have continuity and try to maintain a regular communication update system. Care partners and indeed the individual receiving the care need to be assured on a regular basis that all is going well and that if and when there are changes, they will be kept informed.

A multicomponent intervention for palliative care in dementia focused on the long-term care (LTC) setting. Called 'Strengthening a Palliative Approach to Long-Term Care' (SPA-LTC), it was developed and evaluated in Canada  One of the important aspects of the approach is the educational materials aimed not only at persons living with dementia and their care partners, but also at long-term care staff (https://spaltc.ca/). SPA-LTC includes information on advance care planning because this is critical in holistic and palliative approaches to care.

The US-based resource from The Conversation Project is an easy-to-use tool. It begins with discussing why having conversations about wishes for end-of-life care is important for the person living with dementia and for care partners. It also includes practical advice on how and when to have this conversation – early in the disease process ideally, during moments of greater clarity, and in small, brief, but more frequent conversations. It also includes words that you can use during your conversation together about preferences for end-of-life care. This help can be critical for families who are feeling unsure about how to have these difficult but necessary conversations. The workbook begins with an excellent suggestion: finish the sentence 'what matters to me at end of life is…' (https://theconversationprojectinboulder.org/wp-content/uploads/2016/10/TCP_StarterKit_Alzheimers.pdf). It has additional prompts about how much detail the person living with dementia wants to have and how much they wish to continue to be involved in decision-making. It also has a section for care partners to use as a resource if the person living with dementia is not able to communicate their wishes. As discussed in Chapter 2, many of these difficult decisions are made easier by having frequent conversations about wishes for future care and wishes for end-of-life care.

SPA-LTC includes another resource for families to have conversations with healthcare staff about palliative care approaches (https://spaltc.ca/wp-content/uploads/2021/05/QuestionPromptList_EN.pdf). Asking these questions will help care partners be informed about the approaches to end of life in the setting where their loved one with dementia is being cared for and help to open lines of communication about the wishes expressed by the person living with dementia for their own end-of-life care.

SPA-LTC also has an important resource on how to consider foods and fluids at the end of life (https://spaltc.ca/wp-content/uploads/2024/01/SPA-LTC-Foods-and-Fluids-Trifold-ENGLISH-FINAL.pdf).

Barrado-Martín et al. (2021) conducted a review of the literature on end-of-life nutrition and fluid intake. This issue can cause great angst for families and can put them at odds with healthcare teams. A general lack of education about the needs for nutrition and fluids at the end of life impacted this disconnect, with some families adamant that nutrition and hydration should be supplied at all costs. Even if it meant using artificial means that could impact the quality of life of the person living with dementia (e.g. the need to restrain to avoid pulling out an intravenous line), despite the lack of data suggesting that these approaches are helpful for persons living with dementia at end of life.

The ability to safely ingest food or drink is limited in persons living with advanced dementia and is common near the end of life. For this reason, palliative approaches to dementia care address issues related to eating and drinking fluids. Proper hydration and nutrition are a large part of appropriate dementia care, but at end-of-life care, this issue becomes more complicated (Barrado-Martin et al., 2021). If one cannot eat or drink without choking or accidentally breathing in fluids/food, which is a common cause of (aspiration) pneumonia, hand feeding can persist and is recommended. However, many families wonder about artificial methods of ensuring their loved one with dementia is able to ingest food or drink. Feeding tubes of various kinds are an intervention that is sometimes considered. Putting in feeding tubes can be a challenge for people who are confused, and they might try to pull them out. The European Society of Gastrointestinal Endoscopy (ESGE) suggests that feeding tubes are not recommended for placement for more than four weeks; too many complications from feeding tubes are found in persons with dementia with no evidence of benefit to the person living with dementia (2021). The practice recommendations are not to use feeding tubes with people with advanced dementia. Instead, focus should be on hand feeding and comfort care (Arvanitakis et al., 2021). Food and fluids should be provided for comfort, with a focus on quality of life.

The issues involved in providing food and fluids are complex, involving ethical and sociocultural contextual factors. The best approaches need to balance the advance care planning wishes of the person with dementia, the family, and the cons of using artificial methods for the comfort and quality of life of the person living with dementia. SPA-LTC includes education aimed at families regarding comfort care and approaches to food and nutrition at the end of life (https://spaltc.ca/wp-content/uploads/2022/02/ComfortCareBooklet_EN.pdf). A scoping review of the research on palliative approaches to dementia care found that rural families appeared less willing to use artificial means for feeding and fluids than urban families, but the findings were from very small samples, and any conclusions are tentative.

## WHEN MIGHT THE PERSON LIVING WITH DEMENTIA BE OFFERED THIS TYPE OF SUPPORT?

A palliative approach to dementia care may happen at any stage of the journey with dementia. Indeed, many aspects of the palliative approach to care are best if they happen early in the dementia journey, such as conversations around care planning, advance care directives, and wishes for end-of-life care. These are not conversations that happen once and then are 'done'; it is recommended to begin early and take your time having these uncomfortable conversations. We recommend accessing some resources, such as those mentioned in the first section of this chapter.

There is a lack of information about the 'best' time to introduce a palliative approach to dementia care – all we can really say is that it is best sometime after the diagnosis of dementia. Dementia is a life-limiting diagnosis, and there will be challenges to remaining active and engaged, but a palliative care approach would ideally be considered before any formal care has been initiated. This could include home-based care to help the person live at home for longer, and it would also include when a person living with dementia enters long-term care. Prior to admission to LTC, conversations about wishes for care needs, now that the person is moving from living in the community to a congregate setting, allow for person-centred planning that would ideally address quality of life holistically.

## WHAT CAN FAMILY MEMBERS DO TO HELP AT END OF LIFE?

End-of-life care can feel very isolating for the care partner, and they may feel very lonely if people do not visit. Friends, other family members, and neighbours may not know what to do, so they choose to stay away. This can be very difficult for the primary care partner as they provide increasing support, knowing that the person living with dementia may not be receiving all the specialist support they would like their loved one to receive, and also knowing that the end is near, as they anticipate the loss of no longer having the person living with dementia with them.

---

Carmel reflects on the experience of caring for her mother at the end of life:

As Mum's diagnosis was received at what I now know was a late stage, Mum's progression was rapid. That said, I had the privilege of caring for Mum for three years, but our main issue was having pain relief and determining when she had experienced an UTI. Also, for the last year, Mum was non-verbal and losing mobility on a daily basis. I found the GP to be very uninformed around dementia in general, so we were lucky we had an amazing community nurse who gave us incredible support. I also had gone back to education and had gotten involved in a new cross-border project, 'All Ireland Institute of Hospice and Palliative Care' (https://aiihpc.org/).

This was a life-changing experience. Learning the meaning of palliative care and end-of-life care gave us a quality of life that we would not otherwise have experienced (https://adultpalliativehub.com/stories/carmels-story/).

This led to my involvement in the My Support Study (https://mysupportstudy.eu/), which has now received Horizon Europe funding to continue the project by introducing the training of care home staff.

Grief is complex, and perhaps even more complex with conditions such as dementia, when there is grief and loss experienced both when the person is still alive and when they die (Crawley et al., 2023). The aftermath of the death can leave family members in limbo; their busy life, including providing support and care, now has a very substantial void, and the person who was the main care partner is often forgotten. Bereavement support is very important to think about, and this can come in many forms, from a casual visit to counselling services.

A final aspect of the holistic approach to palliative care described by SPA-LTC is focused on bereavement for families *after* their loved one with dementia passes away. Some aspects of the resources are practical, like what steps to take, and some include recommendations for self-care and provide additional resources (https://spaltc .ca/wp-content/uploads/2021/02/SPA-LTC_Resources-Ontario -2022-trifold.pdf). Care partners can experience a wide range of emotions after the death of a loved one with dementia. Care partners describe surprise at this grief reaction because it is a new level of grief (Arruda & Paun, 2017).

There are many different reactions to death, and the most common is one that causes most care partners to feel shame and possibly even guilt. Sometimes this is a feeling of guilt for being relieved that this is the end of the caregiving journey. Relief and guilt are some of the more complicated emotional reactions, and care partners tend to keep these to themselves, further isolating care partners at a time when they most need the support of others (Stahl & Schulz, 2019).

A journaling approach to bereavement for care partners of persons who lived with dementia is helpful. This tool, called 'Reclaiming Yourself' (https://research-groups.usask.ca/reclaimingyourself/documents/Reclaiming_Yourself_Editable.pdf), honors the stories from care partners who found that an important part of their bereavement journey was to reclaim the parts of their identity that had become care partner for so long. The first section of 'Reclaiming

Yourself' asks care partners to journal about their emotions, and the second section asks them to consider what activities they do to take time out from these emotions. The journaling activity then asks care partners to consider their social supports, and it might be helpful in this section to also consider past social supports with whom care partners have lost touch. The next section of the journaling activity asks care partners to consider the activities they found enjoyable, while acknowledging that many of these activities would have been disrupted by caregiving. The journaling activity asks care partners to make active plans to engage in three pleasurable activities a week. Then it asks care partners how they might engage their creative side to help remember their loved one who lived with dementia. In the penultimate section, care partners are asked to ponder and then detail their regrets in the 'let go of regrets' section. Finally, care partners are asked to cogitate on how their caregiving journey and experience have made them stronger.

Family members may wish to help and be involved as much as possible in supporting people living with dementia, but it is important that they too can also access support and help.

## WHAT IS A GOOD DEATH IN DEMENTIA CARE?

We all envisage a good death (Meier et al., 2016). What this will entail is that, hopefully, our main needs are met, including pain management, spiritual and emotional needs, and dying with dignity in a comfortable, safe place of our choosing with our friends/family near us. Indeed, a review of the scientific research by Takahashi et al. (2021) found just this – being surrounded by loved ones. In addition, however, having one's wishes respected and being provided with care that was person centred at the end of life were seen as important by people living with dementia. This is very similar to the palliative approaches to dementia care described earlier in this chapter.

Phyllis reflects on her personal views about what a 'good death' would look like to her:

After years of working in nursing in a critical care area and dealing with hundreds of deaths, I know exactly what I want at the end of life. My desires are to have my family and friends with me no matter where I am, to ensure I'm comfortable, not in any pain, and not to extend my life with medications. So, when I visualize the room that I'm in, it is a comfortable room with soft music playing in the background, my favourite music, my friends and family all around me. Not sombre, but joyful; reminiscing, laughing, joking. If it's a nice day, let me be outside. I want it to be natural and enjoyable so that the young grandkids can be there and not be afraid of it, so that they learn and understand that this is a natural part of life and it doesn't have to be scary and it doesn't have to be hard. And if it takes them giving me meds to have that appearance, then that's what needs to happen. If the family's hungry and they want to order food, let them do it. This is something that I think would be so beautiful, and it gives the family time to adjust to the loss that is coming. It helps them to become peaceful in the moment and within their own selves as to what is happening. To me, death is not scary. Death is a natural process as long as it is done with dignity and care.

There are many issues to consider in terms of what might constitute a good death from different cultural perspectives. Practical steps to take to ensure that cultural and religious customs are adhered to begin with asking the person, or those close to them if communication has become very difficult. Contact faith leaders for advice if required, and then consider how to implement rituals associated with the end of life of different faiths.

It is important to consider the spiritual beliefs and needs of an individual that go beyond religious observances and beliefs.

Spiritual care can involve not only expressions of faith but also feeling a oneness with the world. Finding ways to ensure that the person can feel at peace is important. This might involve playing certain music, using appropriate touch to soothe, or using scent to create a calming environment.

The other issue that emerges when considering what a 'good death' may entail is assisted dying. This is a topic that can create many different feelings and difficulties in reconciling what one might believe and want for oneself, and what the person living with dementia may wish.

In Ireland, the Decision Support Service (DSS) is a new service established under the Assisted Decision-Making (Capacity) Act of 2015 (Decision Support Service, n.d.). The act is a milestone piece of reform of human rights law in Ireland. Up to now, the two acts of law about decision-making capacity dated back to the early 19th century: the Marriage of Lunatics Act of 1811 and the Lunacy Regulation (Ireland) Act of 1871. The Assisted Decision-Making (Capacity) Act established a modern legal framework to support decision-making by adults who may have difficulty making decisions without help. It means that no human being will ever be made a ward of court in Ireland (White, 2022). When a person was made a ward of court, they were no longer legally allowed to make decisions about their lives. This included everyday decisions. A committee was appointed by the High Court to control the ward's property and money and their overall care. Their personal wishes were completely ignored. Ireland recently debated assisted dying through the Houses of the Oireachtas, and recommended the government introduce legislation (Houses of the Oireachtas, 2024). The Joint Committee set-up to consider and make recommendations have published their report and they are recommending Irish Government introduce ledgislation to allow assist dying in certain restricted circumstances. Ireland is finding assisted dying a difficult subject with which to come to terms. Up to now, people have been travelling abroad to avail of assisted dying, and those who assisted them could be prosecuted here.

Listening to what people would like and finding ways of enacting it will bring peace of mind and a feeling of control over their lives. Although, of course, it has to be strictly monitored to avoid the process being abused.

In Canada, assisted dying is now available in all provinces. Most importantly, it has facilitated people living with dementia to make plans in advance while they still have capacity (Health Canada, 2016; Downie & Green, 2021).

A good death includes the wishes of the individual being carried out, that they are spending their end of life in a place they wish to be, pain-free, comfortable, and with those whom they wish to be present.

A poignant blog was written in 2024 by a leading UK (and international) activist person living with dementia, Wendy Mitchell, as she contemplated her death and her wish to decide when she would die. It was released by her daughters upon her death: titled 'My final hug in a mug...' (https://whichmeamitoday.wordpress .com/blog/). This blog account is perhaps one that brings to the forefront the desire of many people to be able to make an active choice about when they will die if they feel that they no longer wish to live with the symptoms of dementia.

## CHAPTER 8 RESOURCES

We have provided some weblinks in the text of this chapter; other useful resources include:

AIIHPC. (2024a). *AIIHPC launches Voices4Care's book: Positively palliative, stories of care, loss and love.* AIIHPC. https://aiihpc.org/voices4care/

AIIHPC. (2024b). *Home.* AIIHPC. https://aiihpc.org/

Alzheimer's Society (UK). (2012). *My life until the end dying well with dementia.* Retrieved March 31, 2024, from https://www.alzheimers.org.uk/sites /default/files/migrate/downloads/my_life_until_the_end_dying_well _with_dementia.pdf

Dementia UK. (2022). *What to expect from hospice care.* Retrieved March 31, 2024, from https://www.dementiauk.org/news/what-to-expect-from -hospice-care/

Geoghegan, C. (n.d.). *Carmel's story.* AdultPalliativeHub. https:// adultpalliativehub.com/stories/carmels-story/

Health Quality Ontario. (2018). *Palliative care for adults with a progressive, life-limiting illness.* Quality Standards. Retrieved March 31, 2024, from https://www.hqontario.ca/portals/0/documents/evidence/quality-standards/qs-palliative-care-clinical-guide-en.pdf

mySupport. (n.d.). *Supporting care home staff to engage in decision-making with family carers: Scaling up an educational intervention.* mySupport. https://mysupportstudy.eu/

NHS England. (2021). Dementia and end of life planning. Retrieved March 31, 2024, from https://www.nhs.uk/conditions/dementia/living-with-dementia/palliative-care/

SPA LTC. (2020). https://spaltc.ca/

SPA LTC. (2022). Resources on bereavement, grief and loss. https://spaltc.ca/wp-content/uploads/2021/02/SPA-LTC_Resources-Ontario-2022-trifold.pdf

SPA LTC. (2024a). *Comfort care at the end-of-life.* https://spaltc.ca/wp-content/uploads/2022/02/ComfortCareBooklet_EN.pdf

SPA LTC. (2024b). *Foods & fluids at end of life.* https://spaltc.ca/wp-content/uploads/2024/01/SPA-LTC-Foods-and-Fluids-Trifold-ENGLISH-FINAL.pdf

SPA LTC. (2024c). https://spaltc.ca/wp-content/uploads/2021/05/Question-PromptList_EN.pdf

TRU. (2016). *Your conversation starter kit.* https://theconversationprojectnboulder.org/wp-content/uploads/2016/10/TCP_StarterKit_Alzheimers.pdf

World Health Organization (WHO). (2020) *Palliative care.* World Health Organization. https://www.who.int/news-room/fact-sheets/detail/palliative-care.

# REFERENCES

Alzheimer Scotland. (2024). *Allied health professionals and dementia.* Alzheimer Scotland. https://www.alzscot.org/ahpdementia

Antonacci, R., Barrie, C., Baxter, S., Chaffey, S., Chary, S., Grassau, P., Hammond, C., Mirhosseini, M., Mirza, R. M., Murzin, K., & Klinger, C. A. (2020). Gaps in hospice and palliative care research: A scoping review of the North American literature. *Journal of Aging Research.* https://doi.org/10.1155/2020/3921245

Arvanitakis, M., Gkolfakis, P., Despott, E. J., Ballarin, A., Beyna, T., Boeykens, K., ... & van Hooft, J. E. (2021). Endoscopic management of enteral tubes in adult patients—Part 1: Definitions and indications. European Society of Gastrointestinal Endoscopy (ESGE) Guideline. *Endoscopy, 53*(01), 81–92.

Arruda, E. H., & Paun, O. (2017). Dementia caregiver grief and bereavement: An integrative review. *Western Journal of Nursing Research, 39*(6), 825–851. https://doi.org/10.1177/0193945916658881

Barrado-Martín, Y., Hatter, L., Moore, K. J., Sampson, E. L., Rait, G., Manthorpe, J., ... & Davies, N. (2021). Nutrition and hydration for people living with dementia near the end of life: A qualitative systematic review. *Journal of Advanced Nursing, 77*(2), 664–680.

Cox, S., & Watchman, K. (2004). Death and dying. In A. Innes, C. Archibald, & C. Murphy (Eds.), *Dementia and social inclusion: Marginalised groups and marginalised areas of dementia research, care and practice.* Jessica Kinglsey, 84–95.

Crawley, S., Sampson, E. L., Moore, K. J. Kupeli, N., & West, E. (2023). Grief in family carers of people living with dementia: A systematic review. *International Psychogeriatrics, 35*(9), 477–508. https://doi.org/10.1017/S1041610221002787

Davies, N., & Iliffe, S. (2020). *Rules of thumb: End of life care for people with dementia – a guide for healthcare professionals.* https://www.ucl.ac.uk/epidemiology-health-care/sites/epidemiology-health-care/files/demenita_rot.pdf

Decision Support Service. (n.d.). *Welcome to the decision support service website.* Decision support service. https://www.decisionsupportservice.ie/

Downie, J., & Green, S. G. (2021). *For people with dementia, changes in MAiD law offer new hope.* Policy Options. https://policyoptions.irpp.org/magazines/april-2021/for-people-with-dementia-changes-in-maid-law-offer-new-hope/

Elliot, V., Morgan, D., Kosteniuk, J., Bayly, M., Froehlich Chow, A., Cammer, A., & O'Connell, M. E. (2021). Palliative and end-of-life care for people living with dementia in rural areas: A scoping review. *PloS one, 16*(1), e0244976.

Health Canada. (2016). *Medical assistance in dying: Overview* [Education and awareness]. https://www.canada.ca/en/health-canada/services/health-services-benefits/medical-assistance-dying.html

Horton, R. (2018). A milestone for palliative care and pain relief. *Lancet, 391*(10128), 1338–1339.

Houses of the Oireachtas. (2024, March 28). *Press release: Houses of the oireachtas website.* https://www.oireachtas.ie/home

Irish Hospice Foundation. (2020). *Primary palliative care.* https://hospicefoundation.ie/our-supports-services/healthcare-hub/palliative-care-programmes/primary-palliative-care/

Irish Hospice Foundation, & McKeown, K. (2014). *Enabling more people to die at home: Making the case for quality indicators as drivers for change on place of care and place of death in Ireland* [Report]. Irish Hospice Foundation. https://www.lenus.ie/handle/10147/337033

Kaasalainen, S., Sussman, T., Neves, P., & Papaioannou, A. (2016). Strengthening a palliative approach in long-term care (SPA-LTC): A new program to improve quality of living and dying for residents and their family members. *Journal of the American Medical Directors Association, 17*(3), B21.

Kelly, F., & Innes, A. (2010). *End of life care for people with dementia: A best practice guide.* DSDC.

Janssens, R. (2004). The practice of palliative care and the theory of medical ethics. In Purtilo, R. & ten Have (Eds.), *Ethical foundations of palliative care for alzheimer disease.* John Hopkins University Press, 146-156.

Meier, E. A., Gallegos, J. V., Thomas, L. P. M., Depp, C. A., Irwin, S. A., & Jeste, D. V. (2016). Defining a good death (Successful dying): Literature review and a call for research and public dialogue. *The American Journal of Geriatric Psychiatry: Official Journal of the American Association for Geriatric Psychiatry, 24*(4), 261–271. https://doi.org/10.1016/j.jagp.2016.01.135

Miele, F., Neresini, F., Bonjolo, G., & Paccagnella, O. (2022). Supportive care for older people with dementia: Socio-organisational implications. *Ageing and Society, 42*(2), 376–408. https://doi.org/10.1017/S0144686X20000938

Mitchell, W. (2024). *My final hug in a mug...* https://whichmeamitoday .wordpress.com/blog/

Pandpazir, M., & Tajari, M. (2019). The application of palliative care in dementia. *Journal of Family Medicine and Primary Care, 8*(2), 347–351. https://doi.org/10.4103/jfmpc.jfmpc_105_18

Peacock, S., Bayly, M., Gibson, K., Holtslander, L., Thompson, G., & O'Connell, M. E. (2021). Development of a bereavement intervention for spousal carers of persons with dementia: The Reclaiming Yourself tool. *Dementia, 20*

Peacock, S. C., Hammond-Collins, K., & Forbes, D. A. (2014). The journey with dementia from the perspective of bereaved family caregivers: A qualitative descriptive study. *BMC Nursing, 13*, 1–10.

Ross, M. M., Fisher, R., & Maclean, M. J. (2000). End-of-life care for seniors: The development of a national guide. *Journal of Palliative Care, 16*(4), 47–53. https://doi.org/10.1177/082585970001600408

Sampson, E. L., Candy, B., & Jones, L. (2009). Enteral tube feeding for older people with advanced dementia. *Cochrane Database of Systematic Reviews, 2.* Art. No.: CD007209. https://doi.org/10.1002/14651858.CD007209.pub2

Schulz, R., Mendelsohn, A.B., Haley, W.E., Mahoney, D., Allen, R.S., Zhang, S., Thompson, L., Belle, S.H. (2003). End-of-life care and the effects of bereavement on family caregivers of persons with dementia. *New England Journal of Medicine, 349*(20), 1936–1942.

Sideman, A.B., Ma, M., Hernandez de Jesus, A., Alagappan, C., Razon, N., Dohan, D., Chodos, A., Al-Rousan, T., Alving, L.I., Segal-Gidan, F., Rosen, H., Rankin, K.P., Possin, K.L., Borson, S. (2023). Primary care practitioner perspectives on the role of primary care in dementia diagnosis and care. *JAMA Netw Open, 6*(9), e2336030. https://journals.sagepub .com/doi/10.1177/10775587241251868

Stahl, S. T., & Schulz, R. (2019). Feeling relieved after the death of a family member with dementia: Associations with postbereavement adjustment. *The American Journal of Geriatric Psychiatry, 27*(4), 408–416. https://doi.org /10.1016/j.jagp.2018.10.018

Takahashi, Z., Yamakawa, M., Nakanishi, M., Fukahori, H., Igarashi, N., Aoyama, M., ... & Miyashita, M. (2021). Defining a good death for people with dementia: A scoping review. *Japan Journal of Nursing Science, 18*(2), e12402.

Weafer & Associates. (2004). *A nationwide survey of public attitudes and experiences regarding death and dying.* Irish Hospice Foundation. Accessed Sept 29, 2014, from http://hospicefoundation.ie/wp-content/uploads/2012/04/Weafer -et-al-2004-Anationwide-survey-of-public-attitudes-and-experiences -regarding-death-and-dying.pdf

Welsh Government. (2022). *Allied health professionals dementia framework for Wales: Maximising the impact of allied health professionals in Wales working with people living with dementia 2022–2025.* https://gov.wales/allied-health-pro fessionalsdementia-framework-wales

White, A. (2022). Wardship—Adults. https://www.courts.ie/wardship -adults

World Health Organization. (1990). *Cancer pain relief and palliative care. Report of a WHO Expert Committee (WHO Technical Report Series, No. 804).* World Health Organization

# 9

---

# HOW IS IT POSSIBLE TO BALANCE THE NEEDS OF CARE PARTNERS AND SUPPORTERS? LOOKING AFTER YOURSELF

## WHAT FORMAL SUPPORT IS AVAILABLE TO FAMILY MEMBERS?

Although they are never enough, if they are even present at all, and not always around when you need them, the implementation of formal supports by numerous organizations around the world is in place because it is recognized that caregiving is a journey that is impossible to do alone. Care partners can white-knuckle it and avoid asking for help for as long as possible, but at some point, the care needs of their loved one will exceed their capacity for caring without supports in place to help with care needs and keep the person with dementia safe and healthy. Formal supports in terms of residential care, or 24/7 care, are typically provided to families only after some sort of gatekeeping organization has done an assessment and determined that your loved one is eligible for residential care. Short-term or time-limited residential care is also a resource – sometimes called respite care. Ideally, families get in touch with these gatekeeping organizations (in some regions of Canada and the United States, this is called home care, home caring in some regions of Australia, and needs assessment from social

DOI: 10.4324/9781003457138-12

services in regions of the UK) as soon as possible after a diagnosis of dementia. It is possible that these home care assessors won't even want to come out to do an assessment, but it is a good idea for families to know who to call in case things change rapidly in terms of their ability to provide adequately safe care, and this act is one step in the process of planning for the future.

Another formal support, which is, in fact, most families' first point of contact for formal support, is the primary healthcare provider – more specifically, the primary healthcare provider for the person living with dementia. Primary healthcare shortages might mean that many people do not have someone who sees them consistently (e.g. a family doctor), but most medical systems are set up with a primary healthcare provider as the first point of contact, and depending on where you live, this can be a nurse, a nurse practitioner, or a physician. Knowing who to reach out to in case the symptoms of the person with dementia change rapidly is very important. It is important to quickly visit a medical professional if there are rapid changes in the behaviour of the person with dementia, their awareness of others and their environment, or their consciousness levels – this could signal delirium (which used to be called acute confusional state). People with dementia are at high risk of delirium (Fong et al., 2015). Anyone can get delirium – if our body is very ill it can make us confused, agitated, possibly hallucinate, alter the basic attentional systems of the brain, and impact levels of consciousness. The risk of delirium increases with advancing age, and less serious body-based illnesses can cause delirium if we are older, have additional health conditions, or have dementia (Kukreja et al., 2015). For example, a very common cause of delirium is untreated urinary tract infections or bladder infections. Because the cause is medical – and the underlying medical cause needs medical treatment – any rapid changes in behaviour, awareness, or consciousness should prompt families to ask for a full medical work-up for the person with dementia. Delirium is a serious condition and is associated with an increased risk of death (Fong et al., 2015). It is possible that these changes are the evolution of symptoms of dementia, but it helps knowing that it is not some untreated medical condition creating new symptoms.

Primary care providers are also a source of support for care partners. Being a care partner is a superhuman task – at times, it can ask more from us than we, as mortal humans, can provide, thus 'superhuman'. Part of caregiving is dealing with the practicalities of providing physical support for care needs, which can range from cooking, cleaning, and managing the household finances to keeping track of medications, doing all that, and helping with hygiene and toileting. Keeping track of all of these tasks is hard – a lot needs to be done, it takes a lot of time to do – and this will likely drain a lot of energy.

Another part of being a care partner can involve the psychological toll of losing a person as you knew them. Care partners have described feeling, at times at least, like they are caring for a stranger. Love remains, but the nature of the relationship changes. Care partner burden refers to a psychological state of perceiving a task as too much to cope with (van der Lee et al., 2014). On the whole, care partners are more likely to experience negative psychological reactions to the caregiving experience; for example, they are more likely to experience symptoms of depression and be diagnosed with clinical depression (Collins & Kishita, 2020). Care partners do not need to wait to be diagnosed with something like clinical depression to seek help – if they find themselves experiencing a sad mood most of the day every day or they find nothing that they used to enjoy really gives them pleasure – they should speak to their primary care provider, who will assess for other related symptoms that might suggest care partners would benefit from treatment for depressed mood. If care partners have access to a counsellor, a faith-based leader, or a therapist – these are excellent resources to use as well.

Sleep disturbance is common – many care partners lie in bed with one eye open because their caregiving duties do not stop – even for sleep! Disrupted sleep makes all the care tasks harder and makes all of us more likely to be easily upset. Care partners who are having problems with sleep should also speak to their primary care provider. Some care partners are lucky enough to be able to access therapy for sleep, such as cognitive behavioural therapy for insomnia or any dementia-specific sleep interventions (Brewster et al., 2023). Treating disrupted sleep helps make the tasks and emotions of the day a lot easier to manage.

Another major form of support is provided by local (or national) Alzheimer societies. They provide support and education for people living with dementia, their care partners, and anyone else. There are many national organizations (e.g. Alzheimer's Association in the United States and internationally; Dementia Australia; Alzheimer's New Zealand; Alzheimer Society in England and Canada; Alzheimer's Europe) that provide information, services, and support. Some societies have toll-free helplines (see list at the end of the chapter). Care partners do not have to be caring for someone diagnosed with dementia to access their services, and these organizations provide education and support regardless of whether people are diagnosed with dementia due to Alzheimer's disease or any other disease. Some Alzheimer societies offer support groups; some of these are targeted (e.g. spouses of persons diagnosed with frontotemporal dementia) and some are general; some are in person and some are held via video-conferencing or over the telephone; and some support groups are for special groups based on similar backgrounds (e.g. Indigenous caregiver support groups). Some Alzheimer societies also provide one-on-one supportive counselling, and most Alzheimer societies provide education and information. Please consult your local Alzheimer society for their programming, services, and supports.

## WHAT ABOUT INFORMAL SUPPORTS?

Unless care partners are lucky enough to reside in a region with numerous easy-to-access and helpful formal supports (a probable rarity), most care partners will likely rely heavily on informal supports. Informal support networks – more commonly known as friends and family – change in their makeup and how they interact with you through the journey of living with dementia (Dam et al., 2018). Many families living with dementia report experiencing a loss of support from friends and family as the journey progresses. Sometimes, this loss is more subtle – the visits become less frequent or family conversations are now awkward. At other times, it is heartbreakingly clear that a friend has moved on (Keating & Eales, 2017; Lee et al., 2022). We discussed some strategies in Chapters 4 and 5 on how to maintain the social network for the person with dementia and provided some tips on how to keep friends and family engaged; however, in this chapter, we are focusing on the care partner. The reasons for a more restricted friends and family circle are complex, and some are simply because care partners have less time to socialize, or they find socializing exhausting when they finally do it, or they feel paradoxically more alone when they attempt to socialize, or they experience a mixture of all of these (Lee et al., 2022).

Friendships and relationships with family need nurturing to be maintained, and when one cannot nurture these the bonds become brittle and are more easily broken. Time cannot be created from nowhere (as discussed above, the time–consuming tasks of caregiving will likely leave care partners feeling exhausted), which means that relationship bonds must be nurtured using other methods. Less time to connect means that when one does connect, it needs to be at a deeper, more emotional level. This will not come naturally to many people. Care partners can try to express genuine gratitude for the role others play in their life, and state that they wish they had more time to spend with family and friends. Expressing vulnerability also helps to connect at a more meaningful level, but this might not be easy for everyone to do, and, to make this even harder, not everyone in one's social network will respond well to displays of emotional vulnerability.

It is very rare that one person can provide all the support each of us needs from one relationship, and all have likely experienced this over decades but did not know how to label it (Wellman &

Wortley, 1990). As extreme examples, Fred is better at helping with a ride in his truck and will help move something heavy, but does not seem to respond well to you crying. Mary loves to help you solve a problem and is quick to provide numerous solutions to any problem you tell her, but she seems to cut off any conversation when you discuss how much grief you are feeling. Some people are naturally better at providing support in different ways. One of the bigger challenges for care partners who want to make good use of their informal support networks is figuring out who can provide what type of support they need so they can modify who they ask for help with physical tasks, who they ask for emotional support, who is best at keeping you busy and distracted, who is best at making everyone laugh, and who they can go to for anything (a rare friend or family member).

This brings us to another reason for restricted networks experienced by care partners: they stopped contact because after each interaction they felt less supported and more alone (Dam et al., 2018; Czaja et al., 2021). Avoiding these situations is a very appropriate and excellent coping method, but it might be time to consider what we discussed above about the nature of social networks and who does best with which type of communication. Asking one's stoic neighbour, who seems happy to get you groceries if you are ill, to empathize with how you can't stop crying because you were up every two hours the night before, might result in a frustrated social connection for both of you. It would be helpful if care partners knew who to approach for emotional connections and who to avoid having emotional discussions with – aiming for an emotional connection with the wrong person in your network will leave the care partner frustrated and feeling even more alone. Care partners might benefit from taking some time to detail who is in their life and what kind of support they seem best able to give. This is not to say that someone who is always there to physically help them with tasks cannot also become an amazing emotional resource; but figuring out the nature of a social network is a starting point.

Sometimes, people in social networks mean well but cannot give each person what they need, which can result in alienation. Consider a frequent example: a somewhat distant family member sees care partner Emily in the grocery store and asks how Emily's loved one with dementia is doing. Emily is left feeling bereft and upset – she thinks, why does no one ask about how she is doing? This somewhat distant family member means well – they think they are checking in with Emily, but they do not understand that dementia impacts everyone in the home and not only the person with dementia. A gracious response from Emily would be to say 'thank you for asking'. But if Emily were to leave it at that and move on, this will leave her at risk of re-experiencing this pattern of communication that makes her want to cry (or scream) every time it happens. Emily begins to avoid this somewhat distant family member and, if she can, she avoids discussions with them. Understandable. It is possible that they need to be avoided, but it is also possible that this person knows very little about dementia. Emily might benefit from considering if it is worth the risk to help educate her distant family member and state that 'Bob (person with dementia) is doing well, and his care needs have increased – dementia sure impacts the whole house!', or variations on this. Hopefully, with more education about the broader impacts of dementia, this somewhat distant family member might also ask how Emily is doing, but it might take several repetitions for this to happen.

Sometimes, social networks become more restricted because others avoid care partners as they do not know how to help, or care partners avoid others because they believe they don't need help, or some of both (Dam et al., 2018). A reluctance to ask for help is more often demonstrated by people who pride themselves on being self-reliant or by people who had early life experiences where they never had others step up when it was needed (Mikulincer & Shaver, 2019). For these self-reliant people, not asking for help does not give others an opportunity to show them they care. It is possible to practice asking for something small and get more comfortable with asking for more help by practicing this skill. It is helpful for care partners to be clear about what they want help with – this makes it more likely that they will get the help they need. If, for example, a care partner calls a friend who usually provides good emotional support but can move on to trying to solve all your problems when they are stressed – starts solving problems – it could be helpful for the care partner to graciously thank them for their insights and for trying to help, but state that right now they don't need their problems solved, they just need to have someone hear how frustrated they are feeling about their problems.

A final source of informal support for the care partner is the person with dementia who is on this journey with them. Care partners who are more likely to report positive caregiving experiences (an infrequently studied topic in dementia and caregiving) focus on the partnership between their loved one with dementia and themselves, and on fostering the relationship *between* them (Branger, 2019). Care partners who are more likely to report positive caregiving experiences see the care partner experience as a journey versus a nuisance or deviant experience. And journeys are always better when experienced with others. Some spiritual people who have reported positive caregiving experiences describe how their spirituality helps them not feel like they are on this journey alone. Other factors that make care partners more likely to report a positive caregiving experience include feeling you have social support, being medically healthy yourself, having a tendency to practice gratitude or practice acceptance, and being able to recognize that a situation might not change, but your attitude towards that unchangeable situation can change. Finally, care partners who are more likely to report positive experiences in the caregiving journey feel motivated to provide care, either because of general feelings of altruism or because they feel it is their turn to provide care to their loved one who had cared for them when they were children, or some other act that generates feelings of wanting to show reciprocity (Branger, 2019).

## WHAT DOES ONE DO WHEN FAMILY MEMBERS DO NOT AGREE ON CARE PLANS?

Tasks can be hard and challenging, but they become psychologically threatening when people do not feel they are able to do a good job, otherwise referred to as having a sense of self-competency (Stansfeld et al., 2019). Maintaining a high sense of self-competency in the caregiving journey can be a challenging task. One day, handling an agitated moment in a very specific way worked so well, each person laughed and the agitation was forgotten. The next day, these same actions can result in a very different and unwanted outcome. Anecdotally, the caregiving experience has been described as being on a ship, and once you get your sea legs, the ship's waters change completely on you and you have to find your sea legs again. At the core of the distress caused by others judging and even disagreeing with how care partners provide care is the threat to their sense of self-competency. One of the most powerful parts of a well-run care partner support group is the genuine appraisal from others who have been through a similar experience – that care partners did a good job given the circumstances, and that trusted appraisal can help restore a sense of self-competency.

It is very hard to disentangle family disagreements on care plans from threats to self-competence and feelings of being negatively judged. It is surprisingly easy for family members to have all the 'right' answers for how to cope when they are sitting on the sidelines. Only people who are on each care partner's journey with them or who have been on a similar journey really understand what each care partner is going through and understand the lens through which they are making care plans (another reason support groups can be so helpful). Care plans can become miraculously united after full-time care was temporarily the responsibility of the most critical, most 'know-it-all' family member. Transferring primary caregiving responsibility to a family member could be described as an intervention to create more harmony via empathy – caregiving is hard work, no one will get it 'right' all the time, and what worked yesterday might not work tomorrow. Some people will only understand if they have done it, and very few will fully understand solely via empathy. Education on dementia for family members can be helpful, and going as a unit to educational sessions held by the Alzheimer Society or Alzheimer's Association can be beneficial. Care partners might benefit from being open and transparent about their caregiving journey because this can also be a source of education for family members. Parents can express reservations about sharing all the details with their children about their caregiving, particularly if the caregiving is for another of those children's parents (Donnellan et al., 2017).

What can care partners do if they are upset because they feel criticized for their care plans and actions? It might help to focus on a goal of trying to be on the same page, working towards the same goals on this journey. Open and transparent communication, creating a sense of shared responsibility for the care of the person with dementia with them in a partnership, but also in partnership with the family unit, can help create more harmony. Part of open and transparent communication includes one of the most challenging tasks – calmly and clearly telling someone how something they said or did upset you. How is this done? First, this should not be communicated when one is feeling overly emotional – clear communication is best when the heat of the moment has passed. It is helpful to set the stage by asking the person if it is a good time to talk, their answer should be respected, but it might be necessary to re-approach. Clear communication involves telling the person how you felt when they said or did ___. Listen. This might need to be repeated – some people are highly defensive and will deflect or rationalize what they did. Clear communication involves being patient. And once both sides have been heard – it is a good idea to ask how to move forward together with the aim of providing the best care for the person with dementia. It is hard as most humans avoid practicing conflict, but it is a skill all do better with practice, and avoidance just makes it harder to do! Express gratitude to yourself for trying – even if it did not work out all that well. Practice again in the future – see it as a skill that needs developing with practice – a muscle that will get stronger with use. Most of us need a lot of practice at this skill, so don't forget to express some self-gratitude for even practicing.

Despite all best practice attempts, however, some family members will disagree no matter what. Some people will not be able to hear what was hurtful. Limiting exposure to people who are inflexible and do not wish to join in this journey might be helpful for psychological well-being. Care partners might need to practice acceptance of yet another thing they cannot change (in this case, not the experience with dementia but this inflexible, highly defensive person in one's family), and care partners might need to find a way to focus on changing their attitude towards this family member's communications, behaviour, or both.

## HOW DOES ONE WORK THROUGH FEELINGS WHEN THE PERSON LIVING WITH DEMENTIA DIES?

We discussed some issues relating to this in Chapter 8, when we specifically considered end-of-life and palliative care. However, not every person will have been categorized as 'end of life' or given palliative care. In this section, we consider broader issues around looking after yourself when the person living with dementia dies.

How the person with dementia dies will dictate a lot about care partners' immediate grief feelings. Some care partners experience sudden losses due to accidents, some less-than-ideal hospital admission experiences that preceded death and left care partners upset for years, and many care partners observe a death that was serene and everyone who wanted to had a chance to say goodbye. If a care partner experienced disturbing events around the death of their loved one, they will likely benefit from speaking with someone, ideally a counsellor or therapist, about these experiences. A disturbing death will make grief particularly challenging and does not encapsulate the typical grief experience, or bereavement, where sadness and a profound sense of loss are expected because they are unavoidable.

In the care partner literature, they used to discuss anticipatory grief as something experienced during the journey of dementia care (now referred to as persistent grief), but feeling this grief during the journey does not lessen the grief one can feel when their loved one with dementia dies. The death is going to be one of the more memorable grief events in the caregiving journey. Care partners describe surprise at this grief reaction – they say they've been grieving for years, but this new level of grief is different and much more complicated (not complicated grief, the technical term, just complicated) (Arruda & Paun, 2017). For some care partners, they have been able to best cope with the caregiving journey by seeing their loved one with dementia as a different person from their pre-dementia self, and they have not allowed themselves to reminisce about, for example, the woman they married, because they found that it made day-to-day caregiving too difficult. At the time of death, these memories come back and can surprise some at how powerful the sense of loss can be (Peacock et al., 2014).

There are many different reactions to death, and the one that causes most care partners to feel shame and possibly even self-loathing is if they feel any sense of relief. Sometimes this relief is for the end of the caregiving journey, and sometimes it is relief because they felt that this meant their loved one's quality of life near the end of their journey was low and now over. This is one of the more complicated emotional reactions, one that care partners tend to keep to themselves, and helps further isolate care partners at a time when they need others' support even more (Stahl et al., 2019). Sharing a complicated feeling that includes some sense of relief for any reason with others who have had similar experiences can be helpful.

Another somewhat unexpected reaction a care partner might have after the death of their loved one with dementia is rage. Rage because their community has now begun to gather around them to share in their grief, their neighbours bringing casseroles to be left in the freezer. It is not that these wonderful gestures are not appreciated – but care partners can feel rage because they wonder where all these gestures were before. They wonder why everyone comes out to help them manage their grief now, and few, if any, came before, during the persistent grieving. Most societies have cultural scripts about what to do to support someone in their grief when a loved one dies, but there are no such scripts for what to do to help a family on the dementia journey. Maybe it is time we create some scripts.

## WHO SUPPORTS THE PROFESSIONAL CARE SUPPORTERS?

Professionals have access to workplace supports and to other professionals. Professionals who work in team settings cope better because they can share their journey with fellow professionals. The journey is harder alone – even for professionals. Working in the area of dementia care can be hard and it can be sad. It is important to be careful to get help – whether it is self-care or accessing a professional source. Healthcare professionals are at high risk of burnout, or the process of burnout. One of the later signs of burnout is a lack of empathy – human suffering no longer bothers one as much as it used to; you become detached. This is not good clinical practice; this is a sign of burnout (Wilkinson et al., 2017).

Self-care strategies include taking care of one's body, eating healthy and regular meals. Low blood sugar mimics signs of anxiety in the body and can make one feel anxious. Maintain hydration, get sufficient sleep, and ideally get 30 minutes of moderate-intensity activity (you feel your breath increasing but you are not so out of breath that you cannot talk) three times a week. When someone figures out how to make self-care natural, intuitive, and easy to maintain, they should win a Nobel Prize. Although hard to do, everyone has to take care of themselves if they want to do a good job of caring for others, and the same applies to informal and formal care partners.

## SOME CARE PARTNERS EXPERIENCE POSITIVE ASPECTS OF THE CAREGIVING JOURNEY – HOW DO THEY DO IT?

Providing support to a person living with dementia can be challenging, and multiple factors, sometimes known as 'jeopardies' brought about by gender, age, and race or ethnic identity, can all contribute to the sense of burden a care partner may feel about their caregiving role (Liu & Chi, 2020). However, it can also be rewarding, and for many care partners, it is something they choose to do and wish to do for as long as possible. The reasons for providing care may stem from a sense of duty or obligation, but can also be due to satisfaction from the caregiving role and the relationship to the person living with dementia (Quinn et al., 2015). Early research identified hope as a key aspect of feeling able to care and to gain satisfaction from this role (Farran et al., 1991). A strengths-based approach has been argued to be key to enabling caregivers to feel able to provide care, and for spousal caregivers, the ability to find meaning in the caregiving role was key, Shim et al., 2013). In their review, Quinn and Toms (2019) found that the ability to focus on the positive and see the upside of caregiving featured in accounts of the satisfaction or rewards from providing care to the person living with dementia by family members.

In a recent UK (England, Wales, and Scotland) study, a number of benefits were reported by care partners (Quinn et al., 2022). These related to the carer themselves, the person living with dementia, and critically the benefits for the dyad, the person living with dementia and the care partner. The direct benefits identified for carers included identifying aspects of personal growth, seeing glimpses of the person, feeling they were making a difference, and doing their duty. Benefits perceived for the person living with dementia included retaining independence, receiving good quality care, and being happy. The dyad benefit was the continuation of the relationship between the care partner and the person living with dementia. Identifying these benefits was key to enabling the care partner to provide support and care, and is argued by Quinn et al. (2022) to be a missing piece in the evidence base around helping care partners to be able to continue to care.

Clinical anecdotes of care partners who reported benefits included some who felt a spiritual connection to the caregiving duties and saw caregiving as something given to them from a higher power; this works for care partners who are highly spiritual and for some whose experience of spirituality includes religion. Some care partners described psychologically reframing challenges they had experienced in their life pre-caregiving, as helping to prepare them for the present caregiving duties, and this helped them to re-evaluate their life journey more positively. Most clinical anecdotes of care partners who expressed feeling benefits from caregiving shared that they felt a profound sense of purpose in their care and saw it as an expression of love. Children providing care to parents have described the caregiving journey as an opportunity to give back to a parent who had provided them with care in the past. Some care partners have an enviable ability to focus on the positive and naturally see humour in situations that would overwhelm most people, making it easier for them to experience benefits associated with caregiving.

## WHAT RESOURCES ARE AVAILABLE FOR FURTHER INFORMATION?

There are many resources one can refer to when providing care and support to a person living with dementia. The list we provide below is not exhaustive but is a curated list of resources we recommend as a starting point to help determine what might be needed and where support may come from, depending on the country the care partner is located in, because getting information is not always easy, as Carmel reflects:

---

Carmel considers the resources she felt were missing to support her caregiving journey:

We would have benefited so much from a simple explanation of the functioning of the brain. It would have been life-changing if we had been informed of the types of dementia and the expected development of the types of dementia with which Mum had been diagnosed. Additionally, it would have been helpful if we had been told about the behaviour changes caused by frontotemporal dementia.

Family care/support is not recognized for the health cost savings we provide to the state. In Ireland, if you receive a family carer allowance, it is means based and very difficult to access. A good national health programme should recognize and acknowledge the great contribution that families make, and if the carer/supporter is given appropriate support, it will hopefully help sustain their health and their commitment to care for their loved one.

---

# RESOURCE LIST

## INTERNATIONAL RESOURCES

Alzheimer Disease International has a collection of links to national organizations (searched by country) listed in its member associations.

- Website: https://www.alzint.org/our-members/member-associations/

Dementia Alliance International is an organization with exclusive membership for people with a diagnosis of dementia.

- Website: https://dementiaallianceinternational.org/

Baycrest Foundation (Canada) includes links to multilingual support resources from around the world.

- Website: http://www.baycrest.org

- Webpage for multilingual resources: https://www.baycrest.org/baycrest/education-training/educational-resources/dementia-resources-around-the-world/dementia-resources-for-patients/information-in-other-languages

Forward with Dementia is a useful guide to dementia in English, Dutch, and Polish.

- Website: https://www.forwardwithdementia.org/

International Association for Indigenous Ageing:

- Brain Health
  - Website: https://iasquared.org/brain-health/
- Dementia Friends Room Experience will help you recognize the signs of dementia.
  - Website: https://iasquared.org/dementia-friends/rooms/

iSupport (WHO Initiative) is a self-help skills and training programme for carers of people with dementia.

- Website: https://www.who.int/teams/mental-health-and-substance-use/treatment-care/isupport

Strengthening Responses to Dementia (STRiDE) is a project that examined practices, both at a national level and for individual families in a number of countries, to help people living with dementia to live well and to ensure that family and other carers do not face excessive costs that could impoverish them or compromise their own health.

- Website: https://stride-dementia.org/

## EUROPEAN RESOURCES

Alzheimer Europe has a collection of links to national organizations (searched by country) listed in its member associations.

- Website: https://www.alzheimer-europe.org/

Alzheimer Europe's intercultural support developed for minority ethnic groups.

- Website: https://www.alzheimer-europe.org/resources/intercultural-support

Family caregiver support:

- Website: https://www.family-caregiver-support.eu/

There are a number of organizations that provide excellent resources nationally that are likely helpful for people living in other countries. We provide a short list here that is available in English by country:

## NATIONAL RESOURCES

### UK

Alzheimer's Society (United Kingdom)

- Website: https://www.alzheimers.org.uk/

Alzheimer Scotland

- Website: https://www.alzscot.org/

Carers UK

- Website: https://www.carersuk.org/

Dementia UK

- Website: https://www.dementiauk.org/

Meri Yaadain BAME dementia provides resources for Black, Asian, and minority ethnic communities.

- Website: https://www.meriyaadain.co.uk/

NHS England: Dementia care activity booklets are culturally safe activity booklets tailored for people with dementia in South Asian and Black Caribbean or African communities.

- https://www.england.nhs.uk/publication/dementia-care-activity-booklets/

NHS England: What is dementia? A leaflet for ethnic minority communities.

- https://www.england.nhs.uk/publication/what-is-dementia-a-leaflet-for-ethnic-minority-communities/

UK National Health Service

- Website: https://www.nhs.uk/conditions/dementia/

LGBT Health and Wellbeing (UK). Dementia resources for the LGBTQ+ community.

- Website: https://www.lgbthealth.org.uk/resource/lgbt-dementia-toolkit/

National Bereavement Alliance (UK)

- Website: https://nationalbereavementalliance.org.uk/wp-content/uploads/2019/06/Care-after-Caring-for-carers-organisations-v2-1.pdf

### Germany

DeMigranz – German Initiative Dementia and Migration

- English website: https://www.demenz-und-migration.de/en/information-in-english/
- German website: https://www.demenz-support.de/projekte/laufende-projekte/demigranz/

### Switzerland

Alzheimer's Switzerland

- Website: https://www.alzheimer-schweiz.ch

### Oceania

Alzheimer's New Zealand

- Website: https://alzheimers.org.nz/

Dementia Australia

- Website: https://www.dementia.org.au/

### North America

*Resources for African American Peoples*
Alzheimer's Association: Black Americans and Alzheimer's

- Website: https://www.alz.org/help-support/resources/black-americans-and-alzheimers

Volunteers of America Minnesota and Wisconsin: Culturally responsive caregiver support and dementia services for African-American and East African older adults and their caregivers.

- Website: https://www.voamnwi.org/culturally-responsive-caregiver-support-and-dementia-services

*Resources for Indigenous Peoples of Canada*
Anishinaabek Dementia Care

- Website: https://anishinaabekdementiacare.ca/

Indigenous Cognition and Aging Awareness Resource Exchange

- Website: https://www.i-caare.ca/

Native Woman's Association of Canada has resources on dementia care from an Indigenous perspective.

- Website: https://nwac.ca/policy/aging-and-dementia

*Resources for Indigenous Peoples of the United States*
Indian Health Services: Alzheimer's Disease and Dementia Program

- Website: https://www.ihs.gov/alzheimers/

National Indian Health Board: Brain Health for Tribal Nations

- Website: https://nihb.org/brain-health/

The Resource Center on Native American Aging includes a local services locator.

- Website: https://www.nrcnaa.org/

The Healthy Brain Initiative's Road Map for Indian Country

- Website: https://www.cdc.gov/aging/healthybrain/indian-country-road-map.html

The National Indian Council on Aging

- Website: https://www.nicoa.org/
- Telephone: 505-292-2001

## United States

Alzheimer's Association

- Website: https://www.alz.org/about
- https://www.alz.org/help-support/resources is a direct link to resources including for racialized peoples and the 2SLGBTQIA community.

Centre for Aging and Brain Health Innovation

- Website: https://www.cabhi.com/blog/day-1-life-after-a-dementia -diagnosis/

Centers for Disease Control and Prevention

- Website: https://www.cdc.gov/aging/aginginfo/alzheimers.htm

Centers for Disease and Healthy Aging:

- Alzheimer's Disease and Healthy Aging
  - Website: https://www.cdc.gov/aging/index.html
- Data and statistics
  - Website: https://www.cdc.gov/aging/dataandstatistics/index.html ?CDC_AA_refVal=https%3A%2F%2Fwww.cdc.gov%2Faging %2Fdata%2Findex.htm
- Resources for Caregivers, Family, and Friends
  - Website: https://www.cdc.gov/aging/caregiving/index.htm
- Social Determinants of Health and Alzheimer's Disease and Related Dementias
  - Website: https://www.cdc.gov/aging/disparities/social-determinants -alzheimers.html

Dementia Society of America

- Website: https://www.dementiasociety.org/

Alzheimer's Foundation of America (US)

- Website: https://alzfdn.org

- Spanish language website: https://alzfdn.org/es/pagina-principal/
- 2SLGBTQIAA+ resource website: https://alzfdn.org/supporting-the-lgbtq-community-in-dementia-care/

Dementia Connections Magazine

- Website: https://dementiaconnections.org/

Dementia Matters Podcast

- Website: https://www.adrc.wisc.edu/dementia-matters

Flipping Stigma on its Ear

- Website: https://www.flippingstigma.com/

Johns Hopkins Medicine

- Website: https://www.hopkinsmedicine.org/health/wellness-and-prevention/safe-and-happy-at-home

Lewy Body Dementia Resource Center

- Website: https://lewybodyresourcecenter.org/

National Institute on Aging

- Website: https://www.alzheimers.gov/

The Association for Frontotemporal Degeneration

- Website: https://www.theaftd.org/

The Memory Hub (Washington based with online resources)

- Website: https://thememoryhub.org/page/about

Veterans Affairs: Dementia Care

- Website: https://www.va.gov/GERIATRICS/pages/Alzheimers_and_Dementia_Care.asp

### Canada

Alzheimer Society of Canada

- Website: https://alzheimer.ca/en

Alzheimer Society of Canada's Landmark Study uses data modelling to forecast the nation's dementia future.

- Website: https://alzheimer.ca/en/research/reports-dementia/landmark-study-report-1-path-forward

COSTI Immigrant Services. Offers multilingual seniors support, including dementia day programmes, in Toronto, Ontario.

- https://www.costi.org/programs/seniors.php

Dementia Advocacy Canada

- Website: https://dementiacanada.com/

Government of Canada

- Website: https://www.canada.ca/en/public-health/services/diseases/dementia.html

iGeriCare

- Website: https://igericare.healthhq.ca/en

Rare Dementia Support Canada

- Website: https://raredementiasupport.ca/

The Ontario Caregiver Organization has resources on dementia care, including dementia care for racialized individuals.

- Website: https://ontariocaregiver.ca/

The Toronto Dementia Network. Resources within the region of Toronto, Ontario, including day programmes, respite care, formal caregiving services, and dementia-friendly businesses and organizations.

- Website: https://tdn.alz.to

# REFERENCES

Arruda, E. H., & Paun, O. (2017). Dementia caregiver grief and bereavement: An integrative review. *Western Journal of Nursing Research, 39*(6), 825–851. https://doi.org/10.1177/0193945916658881

Branger, C. A. (2019). *Understanding positive aspects of the caregiver experience in dementia: A meta-integration and qualitative investigation* [Unpublished doctoral dissertation]. University of Saskatchewan.

Brewster, G. S., Higgins, M., McPhillips, M. V., Bonds Johnson, K., Epps, F., Yeager, K. A., Bliwise, D. L., & Hepburn, K. (2023). The effect of Tele-Savvy on sleep quality and insomnia in caregivers of persons living with dementia. *Clinical Interventions in Aging, 18*, 2117–2127. https://doi.org/10.2147/CIA.S425741

Collins, R. N., & Kishita, N. (2020). Prevalence of depression and burden among informal care-givers of people with dementia: A meta-analysis. *Ageing & Society, 40*(11), 2355–2392. https://doi.org/10.1017/S0144686X19000527

Czaja, S. J., Moxley, J. H., & Rogers, W. A. (2021). Social support, isolation, loneliness, and health among older adults in the PRISM randomized controlled trial. *Frontiers in Psychology, 12*, 728658. https://doi.org/10.3389/fpsyg.2021.728658

Dam, A. E. H., Boots, L. M. M., van Boxtel, M. P. J., Verhey, F. R. J., & de Vugt, M. E. (2018). A mismatch between supply and demand of social support in dementia care: A qualitative study on the perspectives of spousal caregivers and their social network members. *International Psychogeriatrics, 30*(6), 881–892. https://doi.org/10.1017/S1041610217000898

Donnellan, W. J., Bennett, K. M., & Soulsby, L. K. (2017). Family close but friends closer: Exploring social support and resilience in older spousal dementia carers. *Aging & Mental Health, 21*(11), 1222–1228. https://doi.org/10.1080/13607863.2016.1209734

Farran, C. J., Keane-Hagerty, E., Salloway, S., Kupferer, S., & Wilken, C. S. (1991). Finding meaning: An alternative paradigm for Alzheimer's disease family caregivers. *The Gerontologist, 31*, 483–489. https://doi.org/10.1093/geront/31.4.483

Fong, T. G., Davis, D., Growdon, M. E., Albuquerque, A., & Inouye, S. K. (2015). The interface between delirium and dementia in elderly adults. *The Lancet. Neurology, 14*(8), 823–832. https://doi.org/10.1016/S1474-4422(15)00101-5

Keating, N., & Eales, J. (2017). Social consequences of family care of adults: A scoping review. *International Journal of Care and Caring, 1*(2), 153–173. https://doi.org/10.1332/239788217X14937990731749

Kukreja, D., Günther, U., & Popp, J. (2015). Delirium in the elderly: Current problems with increasing geriatric age. *The Indian Journal of Medical Research, 142*(6), 655–662. https://doi.org/10.4103/0971-5916.174546

Lee, S. J., Seo, H. J., Choo, I. L. H., Kim, S. M., Park, J. M., Yang, E. Y., & Choi, Y. M. (2022). Evaluating the effectiveness of community-based dementia caregiver intervention on caregiving burden, depression, and attitude toward dementia: A quasi-experimental study. *Clinical Interventions in Aging, 17*, 937–946. https://doi.org/10.2147/CIA.S361071

Liu, R., & Chi, I. (2020). Triple Jeopardy? Stress among dementia caregivers through the lens of intersectionality. *Innovation in Aging, 4*(Suppl 1), 60. https://doi.org/10.1093/geroni/igaa057.196

Mjåset, C., Ikram, U., Nagra, N., & Feeley, T. (2020). Value-based health care in four different health care systems. *NEJM Catalyst Innovations in Care Delivery, 10*. https://doi.org/10.1056/CAT.20.0530

Mikulincer, M., & Shaver, P. R. (2019). Attachment orientations and emotion regulation. *Current Opinion in Psychology, 25*, 6–10. https://psycnet.apa.org/doi/10.1016/j.copsyc.2018.02.006

Peacock, S., Bayly, M., Gibson, K., Holtslander, L., Thompson, G., & O'Connell, M. (2018). The bereavement experience of spousal caregivers to persons with dementia: Reclaiming self. *Dementia, 17*(1), 78–95. https://doi.org/10.1177/1471301216633325

Peacock, S., Forbes, D., Markle-Reid, M., Hawranik, P., Morgan, D., Jansen, L., Leipert, B. D., & Henderson, S. R. (2009). The positive aspects of the caregiving journey with dementia: Using a strengths-based perspective to reveal opportunities. *Journal of Applied Gerontology, 29*, 640–659. https://doi.org/10.1177/0733464809341471

Peacock, S. C., Hammond-Collins, K., & Forbes, D. A. (2014). The journey with dementia from the perspective of bereaved family caregivers: A qualitative descriptive study. *BMC Nursing, 13*(42). https://doi.org/10.1186/s12912-014-0042-x

Quinn, C., & Toms, G. (2019). Influence of positive aspects of dementia caregiving on caregivers' well-being: A systematic review. *The Gerontologist, 59*(5), e584–e596. https://doi.org/10.1093/geront/gny168

Quinn, C., Clare, L., & Woods, R. T. (2015). Balancing needs: The role of motivations, meanings and relationship dynamics in the experience of informal caregivers of people with dementia. *Dementia, 14*(2), 220–237. https://doi.org/10.1177/1471301213495863

Quinn, C., Toms, G., Rippon, I., Nelis, S. M., Henderson, C., Morris, R. G., Rusted, J. M., Thom, J. M., van den Heuvel, E., Victor, C., & Clare, L. (2022). Positive experiences in dementia care-giving: Findings from the IDEAL programme. *Ageing and Society.* https://doi.org/10.1017/S0144686X22000526

Shim, B., Barroso, J., Gilliss, C. L., & Davis, L. L. (2013). Finding meaning in caring for a spouse with dementia. *Applied Nursing Research, 26*(3), 121–126. https://doi.org/10.1016/j.apnr.2013.05.001

Stahl, S. T., & Schulz, R. (2019). Feeling relieved after the death of a family member with dementia: Associations with postbereavement adjustment. *The American Journal of Geriatric Psychiatry, 27*(4), 408–416. https://doi.org/10.1016/j.jagp.2018.10.018

Stansfeld, J., Crellin, N., Orrell, M., Wenborn, J., Charlesworth, G., & Vernooij-Dassen, M. (2019). Factors related to sense of competence in family caregivers of people living with dementia in the community: A narrative synthesis. *International Psychogeriatrics, 31*(6), 799–813. https://doi.org/10.1017%2FS1041610218001394

van der Lee, J., Bakker, T. J., Duivenvoorden, H. J., & Dröes, R. M. (2014). Multivariate models of subjective caregiver burden in dementia: A systematic review. *Ageing Research Reviews, 15*, 76–93. https://doi.org/10.1016/j.arr.2014.03.003

Wellman, B., & Wortley, S. (1990). Different strokes from different folks: Community ties and social support. *American Journal of Sociology, 96*(3), 558–588. http://www.jstor.org/stable/2781064

Wilkinson, H., Whittington, R., Perry, L., & Eames, C. (2017). Examining the relationship between burnout and empathy in healthcare professionals: A systematic review. *Burnout Research, 6*, 18–29. https://doi.org/10.1016/j.burn.2017.06.003

# CONCLUSION

This book has provided a brief overview of the journey of living with dementia and the journey of supporting people who live with dementia. We acknowledge that the dementia journey presented here does not capture each individual person's experiences of dementia, and there are numerous personal journeys impossible to describe in a brief overview focused on the typical or average experience. In the book's brevity, it presents dementia from predominantly one lens, which can be broadly described as the lens of majority cultures in high-income Western countries, a model of dementia highly influenced by biomedical understandings. In fact, Chapter 1 was written from a highly biomedical perspective to address the commonly asked questions about what dementia is in terms of disease pathology. There are, however, numerous other culturally bounded ways of viewing dementia outside of a biomedical model. Other chapters in the book, particularly Chapters 2, 4, and 5, consider the day-to-day social worlds and lives of people diagnosed with dementia, and as such draw on a social understanding of dementia. But social worlds vary depending on where one lives and the various cross-cutting characteristics of an individual, such as, age, gender, race, ethnicity, and sexual identity. This book has not delved into any of these aspects; rather, it has charted the journey of dementia and aimed to provide guidance on the typical issues many face, albeit within different cultural contexts.

DOI: 10.4324/9781003457138-13

Understanding cultural views on dementia is important because this intersects with diagnostic processes and is being increasingly acknowledged as an area requiring more careful attention and action to improve the lives of people living with dementia from all cultures. Low awareness of dementia was described across countries (Ekoh et al., 2020). Cultural understandings of dementia, as part of typical ageing, for example, might involve less stigma than can be associated with the biomedical view on dementia; however, on the flip side, this can mean that people struggle longer without a diagnosis and without appropriate supports. Johnston et al.'s (2020) review of research on views about dementia focused, at least in part, on cultures in countries considered low and middle income. They found research on views of dementia expressed by people from Tanzania, India, and China, where dementia was seen as a part of ageing and more likely to be seen as a concern for which formal help was not required. Jacklin and Walker (2020) detailed the different views on dementia across First Nations, Métis, and Inuit Peoples in Canada. Issues related to Indigenous peoples living with dementia include past and present practices of colonization overlaid on cultural context. The review by Johnston et al. (2020) also described views on dementia from global Indigenous populations and found that dementia was viewed as part of normal ageing. In their review of research on Indigenous peoples' views on dementia, Jacklin and Walker discovered many community-level differences in views on dementia, but most commonly, dementia was viewed as part of the cycle of life. Tension between cultural understandings of dementia and the colonial biomedical model was also noted. A review of the cultural views of Black people on dementia from a variety of countries noted that dementia was perceived as a White person's disease (Roche et al., 2021).

Some Indigenous peoples and cultural groups saw symptoms of dementia as spiritual manifestations, such as signs of being closer to God, the spiritual world, or their ancestors (Jacklin & Walker, 2020; Ekoh et al., 2020). In contrast, some cultural views on dementia relate to separate stigmatized conditions or behaviours.

Some cultural understandings of dementia, as part of normal age-ing in the global review by Ekoh et al. (2020), were associated with views that dementia symptoms were not due to an under-lying disease but rather due to 'misbehaving.' For other groups, dementia was the result of stress or lack of social visitors. Some cultural views on dementia see it as a punishment for past wrong-doings, as a sign of being 'crazy', or as a consequence of difficult life circumstances. Stigmatizing views on dementia were asso-ciated with less care, poorer care, or abandonment. The review by Johnston et al. (2020) found that families residing in cultural contexts where dementia was highly stigmatized and associated with shame avoided a diagnosis, did not reveal a diagnosis, or hid away from others after a diagnosis. Recent work in a UK South Asian community found that participants with dementia and their families have 'alternative' knowledge about dementia and do not necessarily understand dementia in a Westernized scientific/bio-medical context (Hussain et al., 2024). This led to misconceptions about dementia and a belief in myths and superstitions, leading people to first seek support from spiritual healers and traditional remedies rather than going to their GP, delaying their dementia diagnosis. A study exploring the beliefs and understandings of the Australian-Arabic community around dementia found help-seek-ing was delayed due to deep-seated family-orientated care norms and recommended that stigma and help-seeking needed to be pro-moted as part of dementia literacy work (Allam et al., 2023).

The stigma of dementia per se does appear related to culturally bound views on dementia, but stigma associated with dementia also appears to be expressed globally irrespective of cultural context. A review of the literature revealed that views on dementia and its symp-toms as negative were present across multiple contexts, and these were associated with self-stigma or the psychological process of internaliz-ing the stigma for people living with dementia (Nguyen & Li, 2020). Anti-stigma interventions were distilled from the literature review by Bacsu et al. (2022). One major category of stigma-reducing interven-tions was educational, including making education in ways that are accessible for all. However, the stigma surrounding dementia in culturally and linguistically diverse communities is a challenge because cultural beliefs, language barriers, limited awareness, and the impact of migration on perceptions of ageing and cognitive decline need to be understood. Additionally, there is a need for individually developed, culturally appropriate services and supports to both address stigma and enhance dementia care within culturally diverse communities (Siette et al., 2023). We hope this book can serve as one such educational model to combat the stigma of dementia. Another group of interventions to combat the stigma of dementia summarized by Bacsu et al. (2022) deserves further attention. These interventions were active and involved contact with persons living with dementia. The components of these interventions included the following features: engaging people with dementia as research partners, participants, educators, spokespersons, and champions to reduce the stigma of dementia; working as a team and treating everyone as equals; incorporating learning with shared objectives or common goals; engaging in experiential learning or learning where you provide a service; integrating relationship building with social interaction time; focusing on the positive rather than the negative; showcasing the achievements of those living with dementia; and demonstrating that it is possible to lead an active life with dementia. This book can be seen as an example of an anti-stigma intervention, and it includes many of the anti-stigma intervention features noted above.

# REFERENCES

Allam, I., Gresham, M., Phillipson, L., Brodaty, H., & Low, L. F. (2023). Beliefs around help-seeking and support for dementia in the Australian Arabic speaking community. *Dementia*, *22*(5), 995–1009.

Bacsu, J. D., Johnson, S., O'Connell, M. E., Viger, M., Muhajarine, N., Hackett, P., Jeffery, B., Novik, N., & McIntosh, T. (2022). Stigma reduction interventions of dementia: A scoping review. *Canadian Journal on Aging/La Revue canadienne du vieillissement*, *41*(2), 203–213.

Ekoh, P. C., George, E. O., Ejimakaraonye, C., & Okoye, U. O. (2020). An appraisal of public understanding of dementia across cultures. *Journal of Social Work in Developing Societies*, *2*(1).

Hussain, N., Clark, A., & Innes, A. (2024). Cultural myths, superstitions, and stigma surrounding dementia in a UK Bangladeshi community. *Health & Social Care in the Community*.p. 11. https://doi.org/10.1155/2024/8823063

Jacklin, K., & Walker, J. (2020). Cultural understandings of dementia in Indigenous peoples: A qualitative evidence synthesis. *Canadian Journal on Aging/La Revue canadienne du vieillissement, 39*(2), 220–234.

Johnston, K., Preston, R., Strivens, E., Qaloewai, W., & Larkins, S. (2020). Understandings of dementia in low and middle income countries and amongst indigenous peoples: A systematic review and qualitative meta-synthesis. *Aging & Mental Health, 24*(8), 1183–1195. https://doi.org/10.1080/13607863.2019.1606891

Nguyen, T., & Li, X. (2020). Understanding public-stigma and self-stigma in the context of dementia: A systematic review of the global literature. *Dementia, 19*(2), 148–181.

Roche, M., Higgs, P., Aworinde, J., & Cooper, C. (2021). A review of qualitative research of perception and experiences of dementia among adults from Black, African, and Caribbean background: What and whom are we researching?. *The Gerontologist, 61*(5), e195–e208.

Siette, J., Meka, A., & Antoniades, J. (2023). Breaking the barriers: Overcoming dementia-related stigma in minority communities. *Frontiers in Psychiatry*, 14.1278944. https://doi.org/10.3389/fpsyt.2023.1278944

# INDEX

Printed in the United States
by Baker & Taylor Publisher Services